T0264237

# Optimizing Sleep in the Intensive Care Unit

*Editor*

KAREN BERGMAN SCHIEMAN

# CRITICAL CARE NURSING CLINICS OF NORTH AMERICA

www.ccnursing.theclinics.com

*Consulting Editor*
CYNTHIA BAUTISTA

June 2021 • Volume 33 • Number 2

**ELSEVIER**

1600 John F. Kennedy Boulevard • Suite 1800 • Philadelphia, Pennsylvania, 19103-2899

http://www.theclinics.com

CRITICAL CARE NURSING CLINICS OF NORTH AMERICA Volume 33, Number 2
June 2021 ISSN 0899-5885, ISBN-13: 978-0-323-81311-2

Editor: Kerry Holland
Developmental Editor: Ann Gielou M. Posedio

© 2021 Elsevier Inc. All rights reserved.

This periodical and the individual contributions contained in it are protected under copyright by Elsevier, and the following terms and conditions apply to their use:

**Photocopying**
Single photocopies of single articles may be made for personal use as allowed by national copyright laws. Permission of the Publisher and payment of a fee is required for all other photocopying, including multiple or systematic copying, copying for advertising or promotional purposes, resale, and all forms of document delivery. Special rates are available for educational institutions that wish to make photocopies for non-profit educational classroom use. For information on how to seek permission visit www.elsevier.com/permissions or call: (+44) 1865 843830 (UK)/(+1) 215 239 3804 (USA).

**Derivative Works**
Subscribers may reproduce tables of contents or prepare lists of articles including abstracts for internal circulation within their institutions. Permission of the Publisher is required for resale or distribution outside the institution. Permission of the Publisher is required for all other derivative works, including compilations and translations (please consult www.elsevier.com/permissions).

**Electronic Storage or Usage**
Permission of the Publisher is required to store or use electronically any material contained in this periodical, including any article or part of an article (please consult www.elsevier.com/permissions). Except as outlined above, no part of this publication may be reproduced, stored in a retrieval system or transmitted in any form or by any means, electronic, mechanical, photocopying, recording or otherwise, without prior written permission of the Publisher.

**Notice**
No responsibility is assumed by the Publisher for any injury and/or damage to persons or property as a matter of products liability, negligence or otherwise, or from any use or operation of any methods, products, instructions or ideas contained in the material herein. Because of rapid advances in the medical sciences, in particular, independent verification of diagnoses and drug dosages should be made.

Although all advertising material is expected to conform to ethical (medical) standards, inclusion in this publication does not constitute a guarantee or endorsement of the quality or value of such product or of the claims made of it by its manufacturer.

*Critical Care Nursing Clinics of North America* (ISSN 0899-5885) is published quarterly by Elsevier Inc., 360 Park Avenue South, New York, NY 10010-1710. Months of issue are March, June, September, and December. Business and Editorial Offices: 1600 John F. Kennedy Blvd., Suite 1800, Philadelphia, PA 19103-2899. Periodicals postage paid at New York, NY and additional mailing offices. Subscription prices are $160.00 per year for US individuals, $576.00 per year for US institutions, $100.00 per year for US students and residents, $206.00 per year for Canadian individuals, $596.00 per year for Canadian institutions, $230.00 per year for international individuals, $596.00 per year for international institutions, $115.00 per year for international students/residents and $100.00 per year for Canadian students/residents. To receive student/resident rate, orders must be accompanied by name of affiliated institution, data of term, and the *signature* of program/residency coordinator on institution letterhead. Orders will be billed at individual rate until proof of status is received. Foreign air speed delivery is included in all *Clinics* subscription prices. All prices are subject to change without notice. **POSTMASTER:** Send address changes to *Critical Care Nursing Clinics of North America*, Elsevier Health Sciences Division, Subscription Customer Service, 3251 Riverport Lane, Maryland Heights, MO 63043. **Customer Service: 1-800-654-2452 (US and Canada); 314-447-8871 (outside US and Canada). Fax: 314-447-8029. E-mail:** JournalsCustomerService-usa@elsevier.com **(for print support) and** JournalsOnlineSupport-usa@elsevier.com **(for online support).**

*Reprints.* For copies of 100 or more of articles in this publication, please contact the Commercial Reprints Department, Elsevier Inc., 360 Park Avenue South, New York, New York, 10010-1710; Tel.: 212-633-3874, Fax: 212-633-3820, and E-mail: reprints@elsevier.com.

*Critical Care Nursing Clinics of North America* is covered in *MEDLINE/PubMed (Index Medicus), International Nursing Index, Nursing Citation Index, Cumulative Index to Nursing and Allied Health Literature, and RNdex Top 100.*

# Contributors

## CONSULTING EDITOR

**CYNTHIA BAUTISTA, PhD, APRN, FNCS, FCNS**
Associate Professor, Egan School of Nursing and Health Studies, Fairfield University, Airfield, Connecticut, USA

## EDITOR

**KAREN BERGMAN SCHIEMAN, PhD, RN**
Associate Professor, Western Michigan University, Kalamazoo, Michigan, USA

## AUTHORS

**GLENN CARLSON, MSN, ACNP-BC**
Division of Critical Care and Pulmonary Medicine, Bronson Battle Creek, Battle Creek, Michigan, USA

**SUSAN L. CAULFIELD, PhD**
Professor, School of Interdisciplinary Health Programs, Western Michigan University, Kalamazoo, Michigan, USA

**ALYSSA CURTIS, RN, BSN**
ICU Staff Nurse, Bronson Battle Creek, Battle Creek, Michigan, USA

**PATRICIA CYRUS, PharmD, BCPS**
Clinical Pharmacy Specialist, Brigham and Women's Hospital, Boston, Massachusetts, USA

**LORI J. DELANEY, RN, MIHM, MN, PG Dip ICU**
School of Nursing, Queensland University of Technology, Institute of Health and Biomedical Innovation, Kelvin Grove, Queensland, Australia; Medical School, Australian National University, Acton, Australian Capital Territory, Australia

**MAYA N. ELÍAS, PhD, RN**
Postdoctoral Research Associate, University of Miami School of Nursing and Health Studies, Coral Gables, Florida, USA

**MELANIE GOODBERLET, PharmD, BCCCP, BCPS**
Senior Clinical Pharmacist, Brigham and Women's Hospital, Boston, Massachusetts, USA

**ANNA KORNIENKO, RN, MSN, CPedN(C)**
Faculty Nursing, British Columbia Institute of Technology, School of Health Sciences, Burnaby, British Columbia, Canada

**EDWARD LITTON, MD, PhD**
Intensive Care Unit, Fiona Stanley Hospital, Intensive Care Unit, St John of God Hospital Subiaco, Perth, Western Australia, Australia

**KAYLEE MARINO, PharmD, BCCCP, BCPS**
Clinical Pharmacy Specialist, Brigham and Women's Hospital, Boston, Massachusetts, USA

**MICHAELYNN PAUL, RN, DNP, CCRN-K**
Professor of Nursing, Walla Walla of Nursing University, School of Nursing, Portland, Oregon, USA

**JAIME ROHR, MSN, RN-BC**
Faculty Specialist II, Bronson School of Nursing, Western Michigan University, Kalamazoo, Michigan, USA

**KAREN BERGMAN SCHIEMAN, PhD, RN**
Associate Professor, Western Michigan University, Kalamazoo, Michigan, USA

**LISA R. SINGLETERRY, PhD, RN, CNE**
Assistant Professor, Bronson School of Nursing, Western Michigan University, Kalamazoo, Michigan, USA

**FRANK VAN HAREN, MD, PhD**
Medical School, Australian National University, Acton, Australian Capital Territory, Australia; Intensive Care Unit, Canberra Hospital, Garran, Australian Capital Territory, Australia

# Contents

Kaylee Marino, Melanie Goodberlet, and Patricia Cyrus

Sleep is a dynamic restorative process that is frequently disrupted in critically ill patients. Inadequate sleep can contribute to delirium and impaired healing. The etiology is multifactorial and practitioners often use a combination of nonpharmacologic and pharmacologic therapies to promote a healthy sleep cycle. There are many pharmacologic agents that may be used to promote sleep, and they display varying degrees of efficacy and safety. The selection of agent(s) should be based on patient- and disease-specific factors. All members of the treatment team can aid in assessing and optimizing sleep for critically ill patients.

Lori J. Delaney, Edward Litton, and Frank Van Haren

Sleep in intensive care is hampered due to many factors; the clinical environment itself exacerbates sleep disturbance. Research suggests that interventions aimed at improving sleep quality have produced positive effects in reducing incidences and duration of delirium. Sleep disturbance is well documented among intensive care patients; however, its prognostic impact is not fully understood. Delirium, disproportionally prevalent among intensive care patients, has significant prognostic factors related to patient outcomes, in which sleep disturbance often is present. The relationship between sleep disturbance and delirium is complex, sharing commonalities in relation to neurobiological and neurohormonal alterations, which may contribute to a bidirectional relationship.

Michaelynn Paul

Obstructive sleep apnea is becoming increasingly prevalent in society and thus critical care practitioners need to be prepared to care for these patients in the intensive care unit. Preparation begins with equipping the critical care nurse with the knowledge necessary to provide interventions which can enhance patient outcomes and mitigate complications.

Jaime Rohr

Patient mobility or immobility impacts sleep. Sleep is vital in the intensive care unit (ICU) for the healing process. Currently, the number of patients mobilized in the ICU is low. Nurses should prioritize interventions for their patients that promote movement. Mobility of ICU patients is proven to be safe and is recommended by current evidence-based clinical guidelines. Despite the established benefits of early mobility, there are potential barriers to its implementation in practice. Nurses need to collaborate with the interdisciplinary team to safely perform early and ongoing patient mobilization despite barriers.

Opioid medications are often used to manage pain in the intensive care unit. Opioids, whether used as recreational drugs or for hospital patient pain management, impact the quality of sleep. Nurses should assess for pain and provide appropriate amounts of pain medications, while minimizing opioid use once the patient can tolerate non-narcotic medications. Nurses should assess the intensive care unit patient's sleep quality and be mindful of the effect that opioid medications have on sleep quality.

Sleep disruptions occur in the intensive care unit (ICU), and pharmacologic and nonpharmacologic interventions can help minimize the effects. A structured quality improvement plan will ensure successful implementation and sustainability of a sleep protocol in the ICU.

Sleep is a vital component of health and healing. Hospitalized patients need sleep in order to overcome their illness, and family members of those patients also need restorative sleep. Nurses can assist with both patient's and family member's abilities to obtain nonfragmented sleep. Education is important for families to understand the importance of sleep, and nurses can also supply families with simple comfort measures such as ear plugs, eye masks, and a comfortable sleep location.

# CRITICAL CARE NURSING CLINICS OF NORTH AMERICA

---

### SERIES OF RELATED INTEREST

Nursing Clinics of North America http://www.nursing.theclinics.com
Advances in Family Practice Nursing www.advancesinfamilypracticenursing.com

---

**THE CLINICS ARE AVAILABLE ONLINE!**
Access your subscription at:
www.theclinics.com

# Erratum

Please note that Pamela Mulligan, MA, BS, RN, CNML, HNB-BC, PCCN should be added as the second author for the article, "Replenish at Work: An Integrative Program to Decrease Stress and Promote a Culture of Wellness in the Intensive Care Unit" by Catherine Alvarez, MA, BS, RN, CNML, HNB-BC, PCCN. This article appeared in the September 2020 issue, 32:3, of *Critical Care Nursing Clinics of North America*.

# Erratum

Please note that Pamela Mullen, MA, BS, RN, CNML, HNB-BC, FCCM should be named as the second author for the article "Resilience at Work: An Integrative Program to Decrease Stress and Promote a Culture of Wellness in the Intensive Care Unit" by Catherine Alvarez, MA, BS, RN, CNML, HNB-BC, FCCM. This article appeared in the September 2021 issue, 33:4, of Critical Care Nursing Clinics of North America.

Crit Care Nurs Clin N Am 34 (2022) ix
https://doi.org/10.1016/S0899-5885(21)00.. .
0899-5885/22/ Published by Elsevier Inc.            criticalcare.theclinics.com

# Preface

# The Importance of Sleep for the Intensive Care Unit Patient

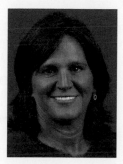

Karen Bergman Schieman, PhD, RN
*Editor*

Sleep is vital to optimal physical and mental health. Insufficient sleep has numerous detrimental effects, including altered immune function and metabolism disruption. Patients in the intensive care unit (ICU) need their bodies to function at an optimal level in order for them to recover from critical illness. Sleep that is fragmented or insufficient can therefore lead to impaired ability to heal and can result in increased morbidity and mortality.

Reasons for sleep disruption in the ICU are multifactorial. Physical pain and discomfort from procedures, invasive lines and tubes, and ventilator asynchrony can lead to fragmented sleep. The environment in the ICU can also be disruptive to sleep. Lights on at night, sounds from people, and alarms from equipment all can interrupt sleep. The bright and noisy environment of the ICU may cause altered circadian rhythms and lead to daytime sleepiness and nighttime wakefulness. While total sleep time may be sufficient due to increased daytime sleep, the fragmented sleep is considered nonrestorative.

Nurses and the health care team can assist the patient to have uninterrupted sleep while in the ICU, thus improving the sleep architecture. Normal sleep architecture requires a sufficient time of uninterrupted sleep in order to progress through the phases of rapid eye movement and non–rapid eye movement sleep. Nurses can monitor sleep, assess for sleep disruption, and implement changes in the plan of care as needed. Knowledge about sleep apnea and plans to mitigate that while in the ICU can become standard care. Both medications and holistic methods can be used to promote sleep, and they are not mutually exclusive, meaning you can use holistic approaches as well as medications if needed. Sleep protocols that minimize sleep disruptions can improve

Crit Care Nurs Clin N Am 33 (2021) xi–xii
https://doi.org/10.1016/j.cnc.2021.03.001
0899-5885/21/© 2021 Published by Elsevier Inc.

ccnursing.theclinics.com

outcomes. Simple measures, such as earplugs and eye masks at night, can assist with normalizing sleep to the nighttime hours as well as minimizing interruptions.

Sleep is a large component in achieving overall health, and with ICU patients, the need for adequate sleep is even more important. The ICU patient's body is under a great deal of physiological stress, and lack of sleep can make their situation worse, while allowing for more normal sleep architecture can improve outcomes. Nurses, being the 24/7 caregivers to patients, are ideally suited to promote sleep and improve the ICU patient's opportunities to heal from their critical illness.

Karen Bergman Schieman, PhD, RN
Western Michigan University
Kalamazoo, MI, USA

9125 West End Drive
Portage, MI 49002, USA

*E-mail address:*
karen.bergman@wmich.edu

# Assessment and Monitoring of Sleep in the Intensive Care Unit

Maya N. Elías, PhD, RN

## KEYWORDS

- Critical care • Sleep • Sleep quality • Polysomnography • Actigraphy
- Bispectral index • Sleep assessment • Sleep questionnaire

## KEY POINTS

- Sleep disturbances are one of the most distressing symptoms experienced during critical illness hospitalization.
- The ICU environment poses unique challenges for sleep assessment and monitoring.
- Methods of assessment and monitoring of sleep in the ICU include polysomnography, bispectral index, actigraphy, nursing assessment, and patient questionnaires.

## INTRODUCTION

Sleep disturbances have been identified as one of the most distressing symptoms experienced during hospitalization in an intensive care unit (ICU).[1,2] Sleep in the ICU is severely fragmented, with increased arousals and awakenings, and with almost half of total sleep time spent during daytime hours. ICU patients experience prolonged time spent in the "light sleep" stage (stage N1), with little time spent in "deep sleep" stages (stages N2 and N3) and rapid eye movement (REM) sleep.[3] Comparisons of normal sleep in healthy adults, versus sleep experienced by ICU patients, are summarized in **Table 1**.

A multitude of factors can contribute to sleep disturbances in the ICU, including patient characteristics (eg, age, severity of illness), environmental factors (eg, light, noise), and treatment (eg, mechanical ventilation, sedation, medications). Sleep deficiency has implications on physiologic recovery and psychological sequelae throughout critical illness. Consequently, clinicians and researchers have developed and implemented nonpharmacologic sleep promotion protocols[4] to improve sleep in the ICU; however, evaluating the efficacy of these interventions is limited by the challenges of measuring and monitoring sleep in ICU patients.

University of Miami School of Nursing and Health Studies, 5030 Brunson Drive, Coral Gables, FL, USA
*E-mail address:* MXE513@miami.edu

Crit Care Nurs Clin N Am 33 (2021) 109–119
https://doi.org/10.1016/j.cnc.2021.01.008
0899-5885/21/© 2021 Elsevier Inc. All rights reserved.

**Table 1**
**Comparison of normal sleep versus sleep in the intensive care unit**

| Sleep Parameter | Normal Sleep: Healthy Adults[38] | Sleep: ICU Patients[19,39–42] |
|---|---|---|
| Total sleep time | Ages 18–34: 6.84 h<br>Ages 35–49: 6.44 h<br>Ages 50–64: 6.2 h<br>Ages 65–79: 5.77 h<br>Ages ≥80: 3.31 h<br>Mean: 6.6 h | Range, nighttime: 4.4–7.8 h<br>Range, 24-h cycle: 7.1–12.1 h |
| Sleep efficiency | Ages 18–34: 89%<br>Ages 35–49: 85.4%<br>Ages 50–64: 83.2%<br>Ages 65–79: 77.5%<br>Ages ≥80: 45.7%<br>Mean: 85.7% | Range: 61%–75% |
| Wake after sleep onset | Ages 18–34: 32.1 min<br>Ages 35–49: 51.1 min<br>Ages 50–64: 64 min<br>Ages 65–79: 77.1 min<br>Ages ≥80: Not available<br>Mean: 48.2 min | Range: 12–204 min |
| NREM stage N1 | Ages 18–34: 6%<br>Ages 35–49: 8%<br>Ages 50–64: 8.7%<br>Ages 65–79: 9.3%<br>Ages ≥80: 27.5%<br>Mean: 7.9% | Accounts for more than half<br>of total sleep time |
| NREM stage N2 | Ages 18–34: 51.3%<br>Ages 35–49: 52.2%<br>Ages 50–64: 52.8%<br>Ages 65–79: 53.3%<br>Ages ≥80: 43.5%<br>Mean: 51.4% | Slightly decreased or normal |
| NREM stage N3 | Ages 18–34: 21.4%<br>Ages 35–49: 20.4%<br>Ages 50–64: 18.1%<br>Ages 65–79: 19.9%<br>Ages ≥80: 19.1%<br>Mean: 20.4% | Marked decrease in slow<br>wave sleep |
| REM stage | Ages 18–34: 19.8%<br>Ages 35–49: 19.3%<br>Ages 50–64: 18.7%<br>Ages 65–79: 17.7%<br>Ages ≥80: 9.9%<br>Mean: 19% | Marked decrease or almost<br>absent |

Normative sleep data of healthy adults are summarized here, based on a systematic review and meta-analysis of polysomnography data.[38] Sleep data of ICU patients are summarized here, based on a systematic review of actigraphy data (total sleep time, sleep efficiency, and wake after sleep onset)[19] and from seminal polysomnography studies in ICU patients (NREM stages N1, N2, N3, and REM).[39–42] Total sleep time refers to total time spent in sleep stages. Sleep efficiency refers to total sleep time divided by total time spend in bed. Wake after sleep onset refers to time spent awake after onset of sleep.

*Abbreviation:* NREM, non–rapid eye movement sleep.

This review discusses and critiques methods of assessment and monitoring of sleep in the ICU.

## POLYSOMNOGRAPHY

Physiologic sleep monitoring with polysomnography is the gold standard of sleep measurement in adult and pediatric patients. Standard polysomnography includes electroencephalography (EEG); electro-oculography; electromyogram (EMG); electrocardiogram; and recordings of airflow, respiratory effort, oxygen saturation, and limb EMG. EEG records the brain's surface electrical activity, electro-oculography records changes that occur with eye movements, EMG records periodic limb movements, and electrocardiogram records heart rate.[5] Standard polysomnography requires the continuous presence of a sleep-trained technician who carefully applies up to 20 electrodes/sensors and monitors the patient.

Using polysomnography, sleep is scored into non-REM (NREM) sleep or REM sleep.[5] NREM stage N1 sleep is characterized by low-amplitude, mixed-frequency EEG activity of predominantly 4 to 7 Hz activity. NREM stage N2 sleep is characterized by the presence of one or more K complexes without associated arousals, or one or more trains of sleep spindles, with total duration of 0.5 seconds or greater. A K complex is a well-delineated biphasic wave, and a sleep spindle is a train of sinusoidal waves with frequencies between 11 and 16 Hz. NREM stage N3, which represents slow wave sleep, is characterized by waves of frequencies between 0.5 and 2 Hz, and peak-to-peak amplitudes greater than 75 μV. REM sleep is characterized by low-amplitude mixed-frequency EEG activity without K complexes or sleep spindles, low chin EMG tone, and REMs.[5] Scoring and interpretation of standard polysomnography requires extensive technical expertise and certification.

Most polysomnographic studies in the ICU have been conducted in nonsedated ICU patients and also tend to have small sample sizes.[6] The interrater reliability (kappa) of polysomnography in ICU patients is about 0.83.[7,8] The reliability of polysomnography in the ICU is further reduced by the critical care environment. For example, it is difficult to remove electrical artifact caused by various equipment used on ICU patients. In addition, polysomnographic monitoring of sleep in the ICU may negatively impact patient care activities, such as frequent repositioning to prevent skin breakdown.

Several disadvantages of polysomnography have likely contributed to the small number of critical care studies. A certified sleep technician is required for lengthy setup, throughout monitoring, and for scoring. There may also be subjectivity when scoring some stages of sleep, especially NREM stage N1 sleep. The numerous electrodes involved in standard polysomnography may affect sleep in nonsedated patients, who may feel constrained by the presence of these leads. Dislodgment also can occur. Finally, the cost of polysomnography is significantly high.

## BISPECTRAL INDEX

The bispectral index (BIS) integrates data from multiple analyses of raw EEG waveforms: power spectral analysis, bispectral analysis, and time-based analysis for suppression/nonsuppression.[9] A patient with a score between 90 and 100 is considered awake. A BIS score of 75 to 90 is considered light sleep, a score of 20 to 70 is considered slow wave sleep, and REM sleep can occur at BIS scores between 75 and 92.[10] A score of 0 indicates a flatline EEG. Measurement of sleep with the BIS does not require the continuous presence of a trained sleep technician. Instead, BIS can be used by nonspecialists. In comparison with polysomnography, the BIS sensors are easily applied and reapplied on the patient, and a screen can provide a preliminary view of sleep quantity. Similar to polysomnography, however, BIS is subject to electrical interference. Some patients may find the sensors intrusive and can easily remove them. The BIS is not recommended for routine monitoring of sleep in the ICU.

There are some limitations to the use of BIS in critical care settings. BIS is an indicator of sedation depth, not sleep stage.[11] When compared with polysomnography, the BIS is unable to accurately distinguish sleep stages. In anesthesia, the use of BIS has been recommended to guide dosage of anesthetics to avoid too light or too deep sedation: the recommended BIS score range is between 40 and 60 during anesthesia, and about 55 and 70 at 15 minutes before the end of surgery.[12] Moreover, BIS scores correlate with neurologic status in nonsedated ICU patients.[13] That is, higher BIS scores correlate with better neurologic function, indicating that ICU patients with neurologic disorders, such as stroke or traumatic brain injury, would have lower BIS values that may not provide an accurate measurement of sleep. ICU delirium, which can occur in up to 80% of mechanically ventilated ICU patients,[14] could also affect BIS scores.

## ACTIGRAPHY

In recent years, the increased availability of actigraphy has led to its more frequent use as a surrogate measure of sleep instead of polysomnography. Wrist actigraphy, a measure of wrist movements (gross motor activity) to assess sleep or wake state, uses accelerometry within a small, lightweight, wrist-worn device that often looks like a watch. Actigraphs can collect data over extended time periods, which can then be downloaded onto a computer. Its software is based on validated scoring algorithms that translate accelerometry data into sleep/wake periods. Validation of actigraphy compared with polysomnography among a variety of participants under controlled sleep laboratory conditions has demonstrated high sensitivity (0.965) and accuracy (0.863) with low specificity (0.329).[15] Actigraphy has also been validated for sleep assessment in healthy infants and children.[16,17]

Actigraphy has not undergone rigorous validation against polysomnography in the ICU setting. Actigraphy tends to overestimate sleep in ICU patients because of inactivity and immobility, especially in sedated and mechanically ventilated patients. Agreement between actigraphy versus polysomnography in the ICU could range as low as 65%.[18] Actigraphy-based studies measuring sleep in the ICU often report wide ranges of sleep quantity. For example, using actigraphy, the mean nighttime total sleep time may range from 4.4 to 7.8 hours, the mean time spent awake after sleep onset may range from 12 to 204 minutes, and the mean sleep efficiency (total sleep time divided by total time spent in bed) may range from 61% to 75%.[19] Actigraphy demonstrates fewer mean nighttime awakenings compared with polysomnography, but higher mean nighttime awakenings compared with nursing assessment or patient-reported sleep.[19] Actigraphic movements have also been correlated with nonsleep critical care outcomes, such as agitation and sedation[20] and postoperative delirium.[21]

Advantages of actigraphy over polysomnography or BIS include its low-cost, noninvasive sensor technology, which does not require the presence of a sleep technician, and can collect data for days or even weeks. Because wrist actigraphs are small, they are not bothersome and are unlikely to be removed by the patient. It is often used for evaluation of sleep-related outcomes in intervention studies, and some actigraphs can simultaneously measure ambient light in the ICU environment. Actigraphy is also feasible for continuous monitoring in pediatric ICU patients.[22] However, actigraphic data should be interpreted cautiously in ICU patients. Neuromuscular weakness, such as that observed in ICU-acquired weakness or neurologic injury, increases the risk of overestimating total sleep time and sleep efficiency. Because ICU patients are often sedated or mechanically ventilated, prolonged periods of inactivity may be inaccurately scored as sleep. Another disadvantage in the use of actigraphy is the risk of removal by nursing staff, who may remove the actigraph during bathing or related care activities, and may forget to replace the device afterward. Although routine use of actigraphy for physiologic sleep monitoring is not recommended in the ICU, its relative ease of use and lower cost compared with polysomnography and BIS make it a popular surrogate measure of sleep.[19]

## NURSING ASSESSMENT

Although physiologic sleep monitoring is not recommended for routine sleep assessment in the ICU, nurses should attempt to monitor sleep by using validated sleep assessments. Inquiring about patients' sleep may serve as a necessary first step to addressing patients' and families' concerns about sleep as a distressing symptom.

Edwards and Schuring's Sleep Observation Tool (SOT)[23] was developed in the ICU setting as a method of observing patients' sleep at 15-minute intervals. The SOT asks nurses to assess patients every 15 minutes as asleep, awake, could not tell, or no time to observe. When compared with polysomnography, nurses using the SOT correctly identified sleep 81.9% of the time.[23] Although the SOT is the most valid questionnaire for nurse-observed sleep quality, it is not practical for routine use because of its frequent intervals. For example, Dennis and colleagues[24] asked nurses to observe patients using the SOT seven times a day, instead of at 15-minute intervals.

Another sleep measure using nursing observation is the Echols Patient Sleep Behavior Observation Tool (PSBOT), which has demonstrated moderate convergent validity for wake after sleep onset and sleep latency.[25] The PSBOT describes four levels of vigilance: (1) awake, (2) drowsy, (3) paradoxic (REM), and (4) orthodox (NREM) sleep. The PSBOT has also been used in pediatric ICU studies.[26,27]

Other nursing assessments have been reported in the literature; however, their reliability has not been reported. Beecroft and colleagues[18] questionnaire included only two simple items: "How many hours did your patient sleep during the study period?" and "How many times did your patient wake during the study period?" Nurses answer these two questions about their patient with regards to the previous night. Beecroft and colleagues[18] did not find a significant correlation between nurse-observed sleep and polysomnography. Ibrahim and colleagues[28] assessment was designed for ICU nurses to visually observe patients and document their findings, such as eyes closed, decreased motor activity, lack of interaction with the environment, and lack of purposeful activity. Yet Ibrahim and colleagues[28] also did not report criterion validity or reliability compared with polysomnography.

Nursing assessment of sleep does carry significant limitations. Seminal studies of nurse-observed sleep[18,23,25,29] revealed that nursing observation tends to overestimate total sleep time in comparison with sleep evaluation with polysomnography. Nursing observation of patients' sleep could be useful, given that observation does not require participation from the patient. However, ICU patients who are unable to move or frequently close their eyes while remaining awake could be mistakenly judged as asleep.

## PATIENT QUESTIONNAIRES

Patient-oriented sleep questionnaires may be a more assistive tool than nursing observation in measuring patients' perceptions of sleep quality. Herein, several sleep questionnaires are described in greater detail.

The Richard-Campbell Sleep Questionnaire (RCSQ)[7] has demonstrated validity and reliability in adult ICU patients to evaluate patients' perceptions of their own sleep, given that the patient is alert and oriented. The RCSQ is a brief, 2-minute questionnaire designed to assess sleep perceptions in the ICU. It consists of five visual analog scales, with each scale representing a different sleep domain. Scores on each domain can range from 0 to 100, indicating poor to excellent sleep quality, with higher scores indicating better sleep quality. Patients are instructed to place or indicate an "X" along each visual analog scale to rate the quality of the respective sleep domain from the previous night. The RCSQ total score is regarded as a global measure of sleep quality. Although the RCSQ is considered the best available option for measuring ICU patients' perceptions of sleep quality,[6,30] the RCSQ can only be obtained from ICU patients who are cognitively able to participate.

The Verran and Snyder-Halpern Sleep Scale,[31] originally developed and tested in healthy participants, has also been tested in ICU patients,[7,25] with limited convergent validity ($r = 0.39$).[25] One study reported that there was no statistically significant difference between the Verran and Snyder-Halpern Sleep Scale and actigraphy-observed total sleep time among acute care patients.[32]

The Sleep in the ICU Questionnaire has been developed to address ICU sleep quality with seven domains and 27 questions, where patients provide ratings on a 1 to 10 scale. However, the reliability of this questionnaire has not been compared with polysomnography. The Pittsburgh Sleep Quality Index[33] is a widely used and reliable sleep questionnaire, yet it was developed in a psychiatric population to assess sleep quality over a 1-month period, and thus is not sensitive to daily variability in sleep.

Although patient-reported subjective sleep measures can provide valuable insight to patients' perceptions of sleep, there are significant differences in results obtained from self-report versus objective measures.[34] Subjective sleep measures should not entirely replace objective sleep measures, but these two could be used to complement each other to measure sleep in the ICU.

## DISCUSSION

The ICU environment poses unique challenges for sleep assessment and monitoring. All of the aforementioned methods have their own respective limitations. How to best measure sleep in the ICU setting is still debated; routine monitoring of any neurologic activity remains challenging in the ICU environment. A summary of the advantages and disadvantages of instruments for sleep assessment in the ICU are presented in **Table 2**.

The latest clinical practice guidelines for the management of sleep disruption in the ICU[35] conditionally states that physiologic sleep monitoring using polysomnography, EEG, bispectral analysis, or actigraphy is not recommended for ICU patients. The rationale behind this recommendation is caused by a lack of high-quality evidence from studies investigating clinically important outcomes: physiologic monitoring has not yet been adequately studied with respect to outcomes of delirium, duration of mechanical ventilation, ICU length of stay, or ICU mortality.[35] Moreover, there is a high cost associated with implementation of these measures.

Although routine physiologic sleep monitoring is not recommended in the ICU, the clinical practice guidelines do emphasize that nurses should routinely assess patients' sleep by either a validated assessment tool (ie, the RCSQ) or by an informal nursing assessment and/or electronic medical record-based documentation.

Future studies of sleep measures should include factors that influence sleep in addition to sleep itself. Studies have identified environmental (eg, noise, light),

**Table 2**
**Methods for sleep assessment in the intensive care unit**

| Instrument | Advantages | Disadvantages | Clinical Application |
|---|---|---|---|
| PSG | Gold standard of sleep measurement<br>Standard diagnostic test for obstructive sleep apnea<br>Can monitor sleep stages<br>Can monitor sleep quality<br>Age-adjusted normative sleep data are available for comparison | Presence of sleep technician required throughout monitoring<br>Sleep technician required to score results<br>Time needed for scoring<br>Lengthy setup time required<br>Requires technician to adjust electrodes if removed<br>Physiologic conditions or injuries (eg, burns) could limit lead placement<br>Interpretation of sleep architecture in sedated patients is difficult | Physiologic monitoring of sleep not routinely recommended |
| BIS | Continuous monitoring<br>No technician required throughout monitoring<br>No technician required to adjust or replace sensors<br>Screen may give a quick view of sleep | Patient or staff removal of sensors<br>Cannot reliably evaluate sleep stages<br>Can be affected by neurologic state (eg, delirium) | Physiologic monitoring of sleep not routinely recommended |
| Actigraphy | Continuous monitoring over days to weeks<br>No technician required throughout monitoring<br>No technician required to reapply<br>Lower cost than PSG and BIS<br>Unlikely to be removed by patient<br>May be able to simultaneously measure light | Nursing staff removal of watch<br>Cannot evaluate sleep stages<br>Periods of inactivity may be incorrectly scored as sleep | Physiologic monitoring of sleep not routinely recommended |

(continued on next page)

**Table 2**
*(continued)*

| Instrument | Advantages | Disadvantages | Clinical Application |
|---|---|---|---|
| Nursing assessments | Easy to implement in routine ICU care | Overestimates total sleep time<br>Frequent assessments are required for optimal measurement<br>Potential risk of missing data because of other patient care activities<br>Nurses may not document accurately | Routine monitoring of sleep using patient-oriented questionnaires is recommended<br>Results should be interpreted cautiously |
| Patient questionnaires | Quick to complete<br>Patients can compare baseline sleep quality with current sleep quality | Patients may lack time cues for day and night in the ICU setting<br>Patients must be alert and oriented (ie, cannot be used in patients with acute or chronic cognitive dysfunction) | Routine monitoring of sleep using patient-oriented questionnaires is recommended<br>Cannot be used in patients with cognitive impairment, delirium, or dementia |

*Abbreviation:* PSG, polysomnography.

pathophysiologic (eg, pain, difficulty breathing, coughing, hunger/thirst), care-related (eg, vital signs, procedures, diagnostic tests, medication administration, catheters), and psychological (eg, anxiety, disorientation, lack of privacy) factors that patients report as disruptive to sleep.[35,36] Assessment of these factors, in combination with a sleep questionnaire, may provide valuable data on sleep.

## SUMMARY

Studies of sleep in ICU patients have consistently reported poor sleep quality. Sleep deficiency may increase the risk of ICU-related complications, such as delirium, ICU length of stay, and mortality.[37] Routine physiologic monitoring of sleep using polysomnography, BIS, or actigraphy is not recommended. Instead, sleep should be routinely assessed by patient questionnaire or informal nursing assessment. Future development of sleep measures, including patient questionnaires, should feature ICU-related factors that influence sleep to best monitor sleep in the ICU.

## CLINICS CARE POINTS

- When assessing sleep in ICU patients, routine physiologic monitoring using polysomnography, electroencephalography, bispectral index, or actigraphy is not recommended for ICU patients.
- Validated patient-oriented sleep questionnaires and/or informal nursing assessments are recommended for routine assessment of sleep in ICU patients.

## DISCLOSURE

This work was supported by the National Institutes of Health (F32NR018585).

## REFERENCES

1. Rotondi AJ, Chelluri L, Sirio C, et al. Patients' recollections of stressful experiences while receiving prolonged mechanical ventilation in an intensive care unit. Crit Care Med 2002;30(4):746–52.
2. Simini B. Patients' perceptions of intensive care. Lancet 1999;354(9178):571–2.
3. Drouot X, Cabello B, d'Ortho M-P, et al. Sleep in the intensive care unit. Sleep Med Rev 2008;12(5):391–403.
4. Hu RF, Jiang XY, Chen J, et al. Non-pharmacological interventions for sleep promotion in the intensive care unit. Cochrane Database Syst Rev 2015;(10):CD008808.
5. Berry RB, Quan SF, Abreu AR, et al. The AASM manual for the scoring of sleep and associated events: rules, terminology, and technical specifications. Version 2.6. Darien (IL): American Academy of Sleep Medicine; 2020.
6. Bourne RS, Minelli C, Mills GH, et al. Clinical review: sleep measurement in critical care patients: research and clinical implications. Crit Care 2007;11(4):226.
7. Richards KC, O'Sullivan PS, Phillips RL. Measurement of sleep in critically ill patients. J Nurs Meas 2000;8(2):131–44.
8. Richards KC, Anderson WM, Chesson AL Jr, et al. Sleep-related breathing disorders in patients who are critically ill. J Cardiovasc Nurs 2002;17(1):42 55.
9. Sigl JC, Chamoun NG. An introduction to bispectral analysis for the electroencephalogram. J Clin Monit 1994;10(6):392–404.
10. Sleigh JW, Andrzejowski J, Steyn-Ross A, et al. The bispectral index: a measure of depth of sleep? Anesth Analg 1999;88(3):659–61.
11. Nieuwenhuijs D, Coleman EL, Douglas NJ, et al. Bispectral index values and spectral edge frequency at different stages of physiologic sleep. Anesth Analg 2002;94(1):125–9, table of contents.
12. Lewis SR, Pritchard MW, Fawcett LJ, et al. Bispectral index for improving intraoperative awareness and early postoperative recovery in adults. Cochrane Database Syst Rev 2019;(9):CD003843.
13. Gilbert TT, Wagner MR, Halukurike V, et al. Use of bispectral electroencephalogram monitoring to assess neurologic status in unsedated, critically ill patients. Crit Care Med 2001;29(10):1996–2000.
14. Ely EW, Inouye SK, Bernard GR, et al. Delirium in mechanically ventilated patients: validity and reliability of the confusion assessment method for the intensive care unit (CAM-ICU). J Am Med Assoc 2001;286(21):2703–10.
15. Marino M, Li Y, Rueschman MN, et al. Measuring sleep: accuracy, sensitivity, and specificity of wrist actigraphy compared to polysomnography. Sleep 2013;36(11):1747–55.
16. So K, Buckley P, Adamson TM, et al. Actigraphy correctly predicts sleep behavior in infants who are younger than six months, when compared with polysomnography. Pediatr Res 2005;58(4):761–5.
17. Bélanger M-È, Bernier A, Paquet J, et al. Validating actigraphy as a measure of sleep for preschool children. J Clin Sleep Med 2013;9(7):701–6.
18. Beecroft JM, Ward M, Younes M, et al. Sleep monitoring in the intensive care unit: comparison of nurse assessment, actigraphy and polysomnography. Intensive Care Med 2008;34(11):2076–83.

19. Schwab KE, Ronish B, Needham DM, et al. Actigraphy to evaluate sleep in the intensive care unit. A systematic review. Ann Am Thorac Soc 2018;15(9): 1075–82.
20. Mistraletti G, Taverna M, Sabbatini G, et al. Actigraphic monitoring in critically ill patients: preliminary results toward an "observation-guided sedation." J Crit Care 2009;24(4):563–7.
21. Ono H, Taguchi T, Kido Y, et al. The usefulness of bright light therapy for patients after oesophagectomy. Intensive Crit Care Nurs 2011;27(3):158–66.
22. Kudchadkar SR, Aljohani O, Johns J, et al. Day-night activity in hospitalized children after major surgery: an analysis of 2271 hospital days. J Pediatr 2019;209: 190–7.e1.
23. Edwards GB, Schuring LM. Pilot study: validating staff nurses' observations of sleep and wake states among critically ill patients, using polysomnography. Am J Crit Care 1993;2(2):125–31.
24. Dennis CM, Lee R, Woodard EK, et al. Benefits of quiet time for neuro-intensive care patients. J Neurosci Nurs 2010;42(4):217–24.
25. Fontaine DK. Measurement of nocturnal sleep patterns in trauma patients. Heart Lung 1989;18(4):402–10.
26. Corser NC. Sleep of 1- and 2-year-old children in intensive care. Issues Compr Pediatr Nurs 1996;19(1):17–31.
27. Cureton-Lane RA, Fontaine DK. Sleep in the pediatric ICU: an empirical investigation. Am J Crit Care 1997;6(1):56–63.
28. Ibrahim MG, Bellomo R, Hart GK, et al. A double-blind placebo-controlled randomised pilot study of nocturnal melatonin in tracheostomised patients. Crit Care Resusc 2006;8(3):187–91.
29. Aurell J, Elmqvist D. Sleep in the surgical intensive care unit: continuous polygraphic recording of sleep in nine patients receiving postoperative care. Br Med J 1985;290(6474):1029–32.
30. Jeffs EL, Darbyshire JL. Measuring sleep in the intensive care unit: a critical appraisal of the use of subjective methods. J Intensive Care Med 2019;34(9): 751–60.
31. Snyder-Halpern R, Verran JA. Instrumentation to describe subjective sleep characteristics in healthy subjects. Res Nurs Health 1987;10(3):155–63.
32. Kroon K, West S. 'Appears to have slept well': assessing sleep in an acute care setting. Contemp Nurse 2000;9(3–4):284–94.
33. Buysse DJ, Reynolds CF 3rd, Monk TH, et al. The Pittsburgh Sleep Quality Index: a new instrument for psychiatric practice and research. Psychiatry Res 1989; 28(2):193–213.
34. Redeker NS, Tamburri L, Howland CL. Prehospital correlates of sleep in patients hospitalized with cardiac disease. Res Nurs Health 1998;21(1):27–37.
35. Devlin JW, Skrobik Y, Gélinas C, et al. Clinical practice guidelines for the prevention and management of pain, agitation/sedation, delirium, immobility, and sleep disruption in adult patients in the ICU. Crit Care Med 2018;46(9):e825–73.
36. Honarmand K, Rafay H, Le J, et al. A systematic review of risk factors for sleep disruption in critically ill adults. Crit Care Med 2020;48(7):1066–74.
37. Weinhouse GL, Schwab RJ, Watson PL, et al. Bench-to-bedside review: delirium in ICU patients - importance of sleep deprivation. Crit Care 2009;13(6):234.
38. Boulos MI, Jairam T, Kendzerska T, et al. Normal polysomnography parameters in healthy adults: a systematic review and meta-analysis. Lancet Respir Med 2019; 7(6):533–43.

39. Parthasarathy S, Tobin M. Sleep in the intensive care unit. Intensive Care Med 2004;30(2):197–206.
40. Gabor JY, Cooper AB, Crombach SA, et al. Contribution of the intensive care unit environment to sleep disruption in mechanically ventilated patients and healthy subjects. Am J Respir Crit Care Med 2003;167(5):708–15.
41. Cooper AB, Thornley KS, Young GB, et al. Sleep in critically ill patients requiring mechanical ventilation. Chest 2000;117(3):809–18.
42. Freedman NS, Gazendam J, Levan L, et al. Abnormal sleep/wake cycles and the effect of environmental noise on sleep disruption in the intensive care unit. Am J Respir Crit Care Med 2001;163(2):451–7.

# Intensive Care Unit Environment and Sleep

Anna Kornienko, RN, MSN, CPedN(C)

## KEYWORDS

- Critical care • Sleep disruption • Circadian rhythm • ICU environment • Sleep
- Life experience

## KEY POINTS

- Sleep is an essential human physiologic need and it is essential to healing and recovery.
- Critically ill patients experience sleep disruption in the intensive care unit.
- Environmental and biological factors impact sleep quality among patients in the intensive care unit.
- Sleep deprivation causes numerous consequences but the link between these and intensive care unit stay is not fully researched.

The intensive care unit (ICU) is a sophisticated environment designed to manage complicated medical cases.[1] Basic physiologic needs such as sleep can be easily overlooked. Sleep is identified as a vital component of the recovery process, especially in those that are critically ill. Sleep disruption among patients in the ICU is a well-known issue. The causes of sleep disruption in critical care settings are multifactorial and include external and internal factors. The ICU is associated with multiple harmful stimuli, such as high noise level (alarms, machines, conversations, etc), persistent lighting, repeated procedures, restraints (numerous tubing, monitor wires), and the critical illness or injury itself. There is a tremendous amount of stress on the human body fighting complex medical issues, such as overwhelming sepsis, severe trauma, and/or extensive cardiothoracic surgery. Patients become exhausted, but it is still impossible to fall sleep because of ongoing machine sounds, lighting, conversations, constant physical discomfort, and a persistent sense of fear and anxiety. Sleep disruption is linked with an impaired recovery process, altered immune response, increased susceptibility to infection, poor wound healing, and damaged neurologic functions and memory. The ICU is a busy environment, where sleep cannot always be the top priority; however, it should be a part of the plan of care.

Faculty Nursing, British Columbia Institute of Technology, School of Health Sciences, 3700 Willingdon Avenue, Burnaby, British Columbia V5G 3H2, Canada
E-mail address: akornienko@bcit.ca

Crit Care Nurs Clin N Am 33 (2021) 121–129
https://doi.org/10.1016/j.cnc.2021.01.002
0899-5885/21/© 2021 Elsevier Inc. All rights reserved.

## SLEEP AS A RECOVERY TOOL

Sleep is a state of physical rest and is an important factor for an effective recovery process.[2] Inadequate sleep in a healthy human is a risk factor for developing adverse health outcomes, such as weakened immune function, decreased energy levels, affected mood and cognitive performance, and increased risk for trauma and accidents.[3] Patients fighting a critical illness need a steady recovery process and adequate sleep plays an important role. Patients in the ICU experience very fragmented sleep. The total duration of sleep during 24 hours period can be normal, but it is highly interrupted, with nearly 50% of a total sleep time occurring during the daytime.

There is considerable information in the literature presenting the evidence that patients admitted to the ICU repeatedly experience poor sleep quality and circadian rhythm disruption.[4] The latter can be described as sleeping during the night and being awake during the light time. It is characterized by the daily sleep–wake cycle, levels of serum melatonin, core body temperature, and many other physiologic indicators.[5] Circadian clocks are present within most cells of the body[6] and it is responsible not only for the wake–sleep cycle, but also it has a significant linkage to many physiologic processes, including the human immune system and the autonomous nervous system.[7] Chronic circadian disturbances carry a strong potential for adverse clinical outcomes and has been associated with increased risk of cardiovascular diseases, cancer, metabolic syndrome, obesity, and depression.[5] Potential reasons for circadian dysrhythmias are environmental and biological factors, which equally contribute to negative health outcomes.

## FACTORS AFFECTING SLEEP IN THE INTENSIVE CARE UNIT

ICUs are designed to provide complex medical treatment to patients suffering from critical illnesses and, therefore, it is far from optimal environment for patients' comfort and recovery. Adequate patterns of noise and light in the ICU should aim in supporting the patient's physiologic functions.[8,9] Nonphysiologic light and noise levels can cause altered sleep architecture. In ICU settings, all 5 senses undergo unusual stimulation and, as a result, patients experience bizarre sensations. The ICU environment been described as abnormally loud, dark, or bright. It is quite difficult to imagine an ICU room without alarming monitors, whooshing ventilator sounds, roaring noise from cooling blankets, ringing telephones, and ongoing conversations of medical personnel. The literature indicates that health care providers contribute to 30% to 60% of noise in ICU.[10] The same report mentions that 34% of noise in the ICU is avoidable and 28% is partially avoidable.

Attaining adequate sleep quality in the ICU is often not a high priority because the life-saving and life-sustaining measures are more important.[11] Nurses tend to underestimate the amount of sleep deprivation perceived by patient.[12] Many disciplines need to assess a patient, and each disruption of the patient contributes to the inability to get long periods of uninterrupted sleep.

There are a multitude of aspects leading to disturbed sleep in the ICU setting. The literature suggests that the etiology of sleep disturbances is multifactorial and can be separated into 2 major categories: extrinsic (environmental) factors and intrinsic (biological) factors. Extrinsic factors presented as noxious stimuli such as various noises, light and medical interventions.[13] Intrinsic factors include the illness severity, anxiety, fear, pain and discomfort. Many of the factors affecting the quality of sleep in ICU are potentially modifiable[4]

## Extrinsic (Environmental) Factors

### Noise

Goeren and co-authors sited Florence Nightingale: "unnecessary noise is the cruelest abuse of care which can be inflicted on either the sick or the well."[10] There is strong agreement in the literature regarding noise as the most common environmental factor related to interrupted sleep. It has been noted that 11.5% of arousals and 17.0% of awakenings were caused by noise.[3] Nocturnal noise levels is found to be responsible for a sleep disturbance in 53.6% of patients.[14] The ICU environment is almost never dark or quiet at night. Previous studies demonstrated that even empty ICU rooms are equally noisy during the daytime and at night.[8] Monitor alarms, medical equipment, and health care personnel conversations reported to be the most common sources of noise.[7] According to patients' reports, the loudest and most annoying noise in the hospital is people talking, especially during the shift report.[10] Patients indicated that they were surrounded by the noise of alarms and the constant presence of professionals.

ICU noise has been demonstrated to have a significant impact on sleep disruption, specifically causing fragmented sleep.[2] Yet, some studies support the statement that noise is not the main reason for sleep disturbances in ICU.[1,2] These sources maintain that the majority of observed sleep arousals remain unexplained because they did not occur within 3 seconds of a sound peak.[2] The same report also presented interesting facts that many studies researching noise level and sleep quality in the ICU are subject to risks of biases. The reasons are the following: the multifactorial nature of the ICU, issues in obtaining consent during a stressful ICU admission, and using subjective methods such as questionnaires. Therefore, owing to these concerns it is difficult to determine the true effect of noise in ICU environment on sleep pattern.[2] Nonpharmacologic noise reduction interventions (ear plugs, quiet times) were found to be effective to improve sleep in critically ill patients.[3]

### Light

Patients in the ICU are exposed to a certain degree of artificial light, which can potentially cause circadian abnormalities.[7] The same authors explain that daylight in the ICU settings is mostly eliminated and substituted with the artificial lighting. The amount of light is excessive during the nighttime. Telias and Wilcox[15] explain that, on a typically sunny day, the light level ranges from 32,000 to 60,000 lux (the unit of light measurement). The same article presents that the daytime light level in ICU ranges from 30 to 165 lux, nocturnal light levels vary from 2.4 to 145 lux, and during procedures lamps can deliver up to 10,000 lux, which definitely can affect a patient's circadian clock. Previous studies found a link between mood-disrupting effects and nocturnal light among healthy population.[5]

Abnormal lighting has shown to have an effect, as was described by patients in the ICU on the phenomenon of time transformation. Owing to irregular natural light pattern, patients were unable to keep track of time while in the ICU. Patients reported losing the reference of the day and night.[16] It was noted that it is common in patients in the ICU to have increased daytime sleepiness. Medical and nursing staff often underestimate sleep deprivation and neglect quiet time routines.[5] In addition, it is very hard to follow quiet time routines in ICU settings, because of factors such as the limited availability of private rooms. Patients reported that the 24-hour activity cycle, frequent disturbances, and variable light levels were very challenging.[17,18] These consistent routines have a significant impact on the sleep pattern and can trigger confusion and, as a result, cause neurologic complications. For example, altered circadian timing of sleep is a key contributor to delirium.[19]

## Clinical Interventions

Medical and nursing procedures is another commonly reported barrier to normal sleep. Several studies demonstrate that nighttime interventions exceed the procedures during the daytime. Patients experience more than 60 interruptions by nurses during the nighttime.[1,20] Medical and nursing activities are an essential part of ICU treatment; however, they provide multimodal stimulation that can result in fragmented night sleep and cause daytime overstimulation. Considering this factor, clustering of clinical care has the potential to improve quality of sleep in ICU settings.[4,5] Some studies suggest that there are hospitals that do not use set protocols to promote a sleep routine in the ICU. The modification of the time for providing nursing care is one of the recommendations regarding improving sleep architecture in the ICU.[21]

## Mechanical Ventilation

Mechanical ventilation has been documented as a separate factor affecting a patient's sleep routine. Aspects of mechanical ventilation that contribute to disturbed sleep are an increased work of breathing, gas exchange abnormalities, and patient–ventilator asynchrony.[20] Intubated patients reported having highly interrupted sleep patterns. They indicated having better sleep after they were extubated, which was also supported statistically.[1] Furthermore, intubated patients were exposed to ongoing alarms, clinical interventions, and a constant sense of fear and anxiety.

There is evidence indicating possible effects of certain ventilator modes on the sleep architecture.[20] Sleep fragmentation was observed more frequently during pressure support ventilation versus assist control ventilation.[20] However, same report further stated that additional studies comparing the impact of 3 modes of ventilation (assist control ventilation, pressure support ventilation and SmartCare) on sleep quality in conscious, unsedated patients yielded conflicting results.[20]

## Medications

Polypharmacy has a strong potential to disturb sleep architecture. Many pharmacologic agents are essential in providing treatment in the ICU.[22] Sedation is a fundamental component of ICU practice and it is required to manage various invasive procedures, to decrease stress and pain, and to promote normal sleep.[23,24] It aims at decreasing stress demand on the body and preserving physiologic body functions. However, certain pharmacologic agents, such as benzodiazepines, do not improve sleep quality and may even worsen the sleep pattern. Benzodiazepines prolong stage 2 sleep and decrease slow-wave and REM sleep.[25–27] Multiple sources support that benzodiazepines associated with impaired neurologic functions (risk factor for delirium), have significant effect on hemodynamic status and demonstrated to have increased extrapyramidal symptoms.[28,29] Owing to its multiple side effects, it is recommended that this pharmacologic group not be used for routine sedation in ICU settings.[28] Many other necessary ICU medications such as vasoactive drugs, antibiotics, and narcotics have been linked to altered sleep architecture.[7,25] They change the levels of melatonin, which is responsible for timing of circadian clocks.

The effects of general anesthesia have also been found to have a connection to sleep architecture. A significant number of patients in the ICU recover after extensive surgeries. It has been documented that general anesthesia has an impact on the sleep process. Natural sleep is controlled by 2 mechanisms: the sleep homeostat and the circadian clock.[6] Anesthetics override at least one of these mechanisms, creating a condition of sleep debt. Sleep and circadian rhythm disruption are often reported after surgery and this aspect puts patients in the ICU at higher risk for negative health outcomes.[19]

Elective surgeries usually take place during the daytime, which interferes with the normal sleep cycle. Poulsen and colleagues[6] presented an interesting report on the differences between natural sleep and anesthesia. When patients wake up, they have no perception of time passing while they are unconscious. It was hypothesized that anesthesia pauses the circadian rhythm. As a result, these authors wonder about additional factors that causes sleep disturbance in the ICU.[6]

Despite polypharmacy and its ill effect on the sleep and neurologic status, many studies support the positive effect of dexmedetomidine.[19] This agent is the most recent sedative to be used in the ICU and is demonstrated to have a more desirable outcome in addressing disrupted sleep. It has been shown to have fewer side effects from the neurologic and hemodynamic perspectives. Few studies have been shown improved sleep efficiency and more closely create natural sleep.[15]

## INTRINSIC (BIOLOGICAL) FACTORS
### Pain and Discomfort

Critically ill patients experience very fragmented sleep when in pain or discomfort. Multiple studies indicate that nearly one-half of patients in the ICU experienced pain all or most of the time. In addition, the patient's pain threshold is demonstrated to be decreased owing to stress caused by noise.[30]

Common causes of discomfort reported by patients in the ICU are cough, diarrhea, muscle cramps, and loss physical activity.[20,22] The latter is associated with greater variations in body temperature oscillation, which has a direct impact on circadian rhythms.[22] During prolonged bedrest, daytime naps are very common; therefore, the patients' sleep schedule can be modified and the patient can lose his or her sense of day and night.[22,30] Early mobilization in ICU settings is suggested to be an effective nonpharmacologic intervention to manage pain and stress.[31]

The critical illness itself contributes to prolonged sleep deprivation.[12] The lives of patients affected by critical conditions are threatened by failure of vital organs and the survival are highly reliant on advanced monitoring and treatment.[16] State-of-the-art technology is the source of ongoing discomfort and anxiety. The everyday ICU experience is routine for critical care staff; however, it is extremely unknown and frightening to the patient.[32] Therefore, the value of comfort and empathy from medical personnel cannot be overstated.[32]

### Stress and Anxiety

Stress and anxiety cannot be ignored as contributing factors to sleep disturbances in the ICU. A strong emotional response is to be expected in patients admitted to the ICU and needs to be mitigated.[32] Critical conditions occur in a sudden and unforeseen way and they often present as situations of great distress and despair. Oftentimes patients admitted to the ICU wake up in absolute fear, not able to understand what is happening to them. Patients in the ICU reported a constant sense of anxiety, bizarre feelings, and threat of death.[1] They are subject to constant stimuli that might alter their sleep and neurocognitive perceptions.[30]

Anxiety is documented to be aggravated by environmental factors such as noise and light.[30] Patients expressed that alarm noises and various intensity lights make to alter their senses and to cause delusions. Patients described nighttime as a very frightening experience because of the ongoing presence of disturbing hallucinations. Patients reported being afraid to fall asleep because they will lose control over themselves and vivid nightmares will exacerbate their fears.[16] They can be afraid that they will never be able to open their eyes or see their loved ones. Patients treated in ICU have very limited personal control; they often have difficulties in communicating with health care professionals and often are unable advocate for themselves.[17]

Statistical data and patients' reports regarding stressors affecting sleep in ICU were analyzed and summarized in this sections. However, the existence of peer-reviewed patient-focused research was found to be scarce. Analysis of patient self-reports was restricted to few studies owing to minimal availability. Patients treated in ICU have limited competencies to provide responses owing to presence of cognitive abilities and levels of alertness.

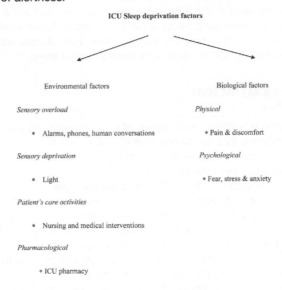

## SUMMARY

Sleep is basic human need and is vital component for healing and restoration processes. Numerous studies indicate that patients in the ICU experience substantial sleep disruption. Patients rely on advanced technology to recover from complex health conditions. Extremely dynamic and complex ICU is not an ideal environment for a good sleep quality. Current research supports the idea that there is a negative impact of the ICU environment on sleep architecture. Evidence shows that multiple environmental and biological factors can potentially cause disrupted sleep in the ICU. Noise and light have been the most commonly documented environmental factors affecting critically ill patients. Multiple studies focus on analyzing the noise as a factor and how it impacts sleep quality in ICU. Despite it being a major factor for disrupted sleep, studies do not support the statement that noise is solely accountable for sleep disturbances. The underlying pathophysiology of the critical illness is also a significant determinant for low sleep quality; acutely ill patients require frequent monitoring and aggressive treatment. There is strong link between clinical interventions and sleep architecture. It has been documented that both sleep consolidation and circadian timing of sleep were disrupted in patients postoperatively.[19]

There is a strong correlation between all these factors and no single factor is entirely the responsible for disrupted sleep in the ICU. Critically ill patients are exposed to multiple intrinsic and extrinsic factors; some factors can be controlled and some cannot. Sleep disturbances are multifactorial owing to the busy, multidisciplinary ICU environment.

A lack of adequate sleep has a strong potential to put critically ill patients at risk for increased morbidity and mortality. Sleep deprivation increases risk for hypertension, diabetes mellitus, infections, adverse neurologic functions, and increased hospital length of stay.

## CLINICAL RELEVANCE

The common themes of research related to ICU environment and sleep quality are the presence of numerous strategies and suggestions to address this matter. Hospitals implement different methods targeting all possible factors that impact sleep quality. For example, initiating novel pharmacologic and nursing interventions. Despite of these initiatives the problem of poor sleep quality remains to be very relevant in ICU.

Sleep disruption is influenced by numerous factors that undergo constant change in dynamic ICU environment. Further research is needed in health care to address the needs of the critically ill, including limiting the environment's impact on sleep. Any proposed interventions to address sleep disturbances in ICU also should be multifactorial and need to be balanced between safety and clinical activities.[4]

## CLINICS CARE POINTS

- Sleep is an essential human physiologic need and it is an imperative component in facilitating recovery from disease. Sleep is often overlooked in the ICU as a low priority item for patients undergoing treatment for acute illnesses.

- Critically ill patients experience sleep disruption to a significant extent. The quantity of sleep is unaffected, but sleep quality is grossly compromised. Patients who have been discharged from the ICU reported highly fragmented sleep while recovering from critical illness, which limits a patient's ability to restore physiologic and cognitive functions.

- Environmental (noise and light) and biological (critical illness) factors contribute to poor sleep quality in the ICU. Our understanding the interaction of these factors is incomplete; however, it is known that there is no single factor is solely responsible for the fragmented sleep experienced in the ICU. The critical care field is very complex and ever evolving. Therefore, research about sleep and the ICU environment needs to be ongoing; strategies to address sleep deprivation in the ICU should be multifactorial.

- Sleep deprivation causes numerous consequences on healthy individuals, but the link between these factors and the ICU is not understood fully. The impact of disturbed sleep on length of ICU stay, mechanical ventilation weaning, hospital-associated morbidity, and mortality needs to be investigated further.

## DISCLOSURE

The author has nothing to disclose.

## REFERENCES

1. Alsulami G, Rice AM, Kidd L. Prospective repeated assessment of self-reported sleep quality and sleep disruptive factors in the intensive care unit: acceptability of daily assessment of sleep quality. BMJ Open 2019;9(6). https://doi.org/10.

1136/bmjopen-2019-029957. Available at: https://search.proquest.com/docview/2244002888?accountid=26389.

2. Horsten S, Reinke L, Absalom AR, et al. Systematic review of the effects of intensive-care-unit noise on sleep of healthy subjects and the critically ill. Br J Anaesth 2018;120:443–52.

3. Boyko Y, Jennum P, Nikolic M, et al. Sleep in intensive care unit: the role of environment. J Crit Care 2017;37:99–105.

4. Stewart JA, Green C, Stewart J, et al. Factors influencing quality of sleep among non-mechanically ventilated patients in the Intensive Care Unit. Aust Crit Care 2017;30:85–90.

5. Oldham MA, Lee HB, Desan PH. Circadian rhythm disruption in the critically ill: an opportunity for improving outcomes. Crit Care Med 2016;44:207–17.

6. Poulsen RC, Warman GR, Sleigh J, et al. How does general anaesthesia affect the circadian clock? Sleep Med Rev 2016;2018(37):35–44.

7. Korompeli A, Muurlink O, Kavrochorianou N, et al. Circadian disruption of ICU patients: a review of pathways, expression and interventions. J Crit Care 2016; 2017(38):269–77.

8. Voigt LP, Reynolds K, Mehryar M, et al. Monitoring sound and light continuously in an intensive care unit patient room: a pilot study. J Crit Care 2016;2017(39):36.

9. Prajapat B, Sandhya AS, Chaudhry D. Evaluation of sleep and factors affecting it in patients recovering in intensive care units (ICU) and step down units(SDU). Sleep Med 2017;40:e268.

10. Goeren D, John S, Meskill K, et al. Quiet time: a noise reduction initiative in a neurosurgical intensive care unit. Crit Care Nurse 2018;38:38–44.

11. Walter E. See no lights, hear no alarms: sleeping in the ICU. Crit Care Alert 2015;23(4):25–6. Available at: https://search.proquest.com/docview/1987263379?accountid=26389.

12. Grimm J. Sleep deprivation in the intensive care patient. Crit Care Nurse 2020;40:e16–24.

13. Delaney LJ, Currie MJ, Huang HC, et al. Investigating the application of motion accelerometers as a sleep monitoring technique and the clinical burden of the intensive care environment on sleep quality: study protocol for a prospective observational study in Australia. BMJ Open 2018;8(1). https://doi.org/10.1136/bmjopen-2017-019704. Available at: https://search.proquest.com/docview/2099470896?accountid=26389.

14. Bani Younis M, Hayajneh FA. Quality of sleep among intensive care unit patients: a literature review. Crit Care Nurs Q 2018;41:170–7.

15. Telias I, Wilcox ME. Sleep and circadian rhythm in critical illness. Crit Care 2019; 23:82.

16. da Cruz de Castro CMSP, Rebelo Botelho MA. The experience of the persons with critical condition hospitalized in an intensive care unit. J Nurs UFPE. 2017;11(9):3386–94.

17. Darbyshire JL, Greig PR, Vollam S, et al. "I can remember sort of vivid People…but to me they were plasticine." delusions on the intensive care unit: what do patients think is going on? PLoS One 2016;11(4). https://doi.org/10.1371/journal.pone.0153775. Available at: https://search.proquest.com/docview/1782829991?accountid=26389.

18. Caruana N, MSN RN, McKinley S, et al. Sleep quality during and after cardiothoracic intensive care and psychological health during recovery. J Cardiovasc Nurs 2018;33(4):E40–9.

19. Lu Y, Li Y, Wang L, et al. Promoting sleep and circadian health may prevent post-operative delirium: a systematic review and meta-analysis of randomized clinical trials. Sleep Med Rev 2019;48:101207.
20. Al Mutair M, Shamsan A, Abbas S, et al. Sleep deprivation etiologies among patients in the intensive care unit: literature review. Dimens Crit Care Nurs 2020; 39(4):203–10.
21. Bani Younis M, Hayajneh F, Batiha A. Measurement and nonpharmacologic management of sleep disturbance in the intensive care units: a literature review. Crit Care Nurs Q 2019;42:75–80.
22. Drouot X, Quentin S. Sleep neurobiology and critical care illness. Crit Care Clin 2015;31:379–91.
23. Halpin E, Inch H, O'Neill M. Dexmedetomidine's relationship to delirium in patients undergoing cardiac surgery: a systematic review. Crit Care Nurs Q 2020; 43:28–38.
24. Morgan D, Tsai SC. Sleep and the endocrine system. Crit Care Clin 2015;31: 403–18.
25. McFeely J. Patients rarely sleep in the ICU. Crit Care alert 2016;24:17–9.
26. Wåhlin I, Samuelsson P, Ågren S. What do patients rate as most important when cared for in the ICU and how often is this met? – an empowerment questionnaire survey. J Crit Care 2017;40:83–90.
27. Beltrami FG, Nguyen XL, Pichereau C, et al. Sleep in the intensive care unit. J Bras Pneumol 2015;41(6):539–46.
28. Fontaine GV, Der Nigoghossian C, Hamilton LA. Melatonin, ramelteon, suvorexant, and dexmedetomidine to promote sleep and prevent delirium In critically ill patients: a narrative review with practical applications. Crit Care Nurs Q 2020; 43:232–50.
29. Yang C, Tseng P, Pei-Chen Chang J, et al. Melatonergic agents in the prevention of delirium: a network meta-analysis of randomized controlled trials. Sleep Med Rev 2020;50:101235.
30. Pisani MA, Friese RS, Gehlbach BK, et al. Sleep in the intensive care unit. Am J Respir Crit Care Med 2015;191(7):731–8. Available at: https://search.proquest.com/docview/1670195845?accountid=26389.
31. Rivosecchi RM, Smithburger PL, Svec S, et al. Nonpharmacological interventions to prevent delirium: an evidence-based systematic review. Crit Care Nurse 2015; 35:39–49.
32. Shapiro PA. Psychiatric aspects of heart disease (and cardiac aspects of psychiatric disease) in critical care. Crit Care Clin 2017;33:619–34.

# Holistic Approaches to Support Sleep in the Intensive Care Unit Patient

Lisa R. Singleterry, PhD, RN, CNE[a],*, Susan L. Caulfield, PhD[b]

## KEYWORDS

- Holistic approaches • Sleep • Intensive care unit (ICU)

## KEY POINTS

- Holistic approaches should be considered for integrative practice to improve sleep in the intensive care unit (ICU).
- Independent nursing actions include holistic approaches that can support an optimal healing environment and should be considered when developing a sleep protocol.
- Aromatherapy, guided imagery, and mindfulness can be easily employed by ICU nurses.

## INTRODUCTION/HISTORY/DEFINITIONS/BACKGROUND

Seven to 8 hours of sleep is considered adequate and roughly 60% of those surveyed in the United States between 2004 and 2017 reported getting adequate sleep.[1] During this time, there was a 4% increase in the number of US adults who report getting 6 hours or less of sleep. This translates to approximately 44% of the US population having a history of inadequate sleep. Inadequate sleep can have physiologic effects on the immune system, hormone levels, pulmonary mechanics, and neuro-cognition,[2,3] and in the hospital, contribute to intensive care unit (ICU) delirium and prolonged mechanical ventilation.[4] Hospitalized people have multiple environmental and care-related factors that can disturb sleep, such as noise, lighting practices, patient care activities, diagnostic procedures, and the use of sedatives and analgesics.[2,5,6] Further, people admitted to an ICU can have profound pathophysiological factors such as organ dysfunction, inflammatory response, pain, and psychosis making them even more vulnerable to inadequate sleep or sleep disturbance/disruption, ultimately producing physiologic effects that can impact patient outcomes.

Medically focused practices in the acute care hospital setting can be augmented by nursing practices that focus on interpersonal, emotional, and spiritual needs that

[a] Bronson School of Nursing, Western Michigan University, 1903 W. Michigan Avenue, Kalamazoo, MI 49008, USA; [b] School of Interdisciplinary Health Programs, Western Michigan University, 1903 W. Michigan Avenue, Kalamazoo, MI 49008, USA
* Corresponding author.
E-mail address: lisa.singleterry@wmich.edu

Crit Care Nurs Clin N Am 33 (2021) 131–144
https://doi.org/10.1016/j.cnc.2021.01.005
0899-5885/21/© 2021 Elsevier Inc. All rights reserved.

ccnursing.theclinics.com

improve comfort[7,8] and sleep in the ICU patient.[9] Altman and colleagues[9] conducted a systematic review that focused on sleep disturbance post-hospitalization, wherein they recognized the interrelatedness of sleep patterns before hospitalization, during hospitalization, and post-hospitalization. Recognizing this, teaching and learning approaches to augment sleep will involve internal, interpersonal, behavioral, and external factors.[10] Using the foundation of Optimal Healing Environments[10] this article reviews and suggests holistic approaches that should be considered as integrative care and included in unit protocols to help with sleep in the ICU patient.

## SLEEP QUALITY

Sleep quality can be measured in several ways, from a simple equation of how many hours one spent in bed, subtracting for time it took to fall asleep and time awake during the night, to more elaborate indices such as the Pittsburgh Sleep Quality Index (PSQI).[11] One of the issues that arises in systematic reviews of sleep and hospitalized patients is the various ways in which sleep is defined and measured. Narrowing the scope of that is beyond the work of this article, but needs to be acknowledged given the multiple ways in which sleep is measured throughout the extant research. The sleep issue is labeled as sleep quality, sleep disruption, sleep disturbance, and other variations, such as total sleep time, time to sleep, and sleep-onset latency. Throughout the article, we use the term sleep quality as the overriding concern.

Sleep is listed as a base element on the Maslow hierarchy under physiologic needs. Maslow[12] described these physiologic needs as automatic, and they are often ignored until there is a disruption. Normal sleep patterns include 2 major categories: rapid eye movement (REM) and non-REM (NREM), where NREM is further subdivided into 3 stages (N1–3). Devlin and colleagues[4] characterized sleep disruption as lengthening of N1 and N2 (light sleep), a decrease in both REM and N3 (slow-wave) sleep, and circadian rhythm changes. These changes are not easily assessed by a nurse, as total observable sleep time may appear normal. Sleep disturbance also may occur because a patient's condition in the ICU setting needs care that includes several arousals or awakenings per hour, the person may be mechanically ventilated, and/or receiving opioid analgesic and amnesic-inducing medications. Environmental factors such as noise, light, room ventilation, and bad odors; physiologic factors such as pain, difficulty breathing, nausea, and need to urinate/defecate; and psychological factors such as worry, fear, and loneliness also play a role in sleep disruption.[2] Given all these factors that can disrupt sleep in the ICU, it is not surprising that sleep is considered to be one of the most common stressors in the ICU. Indeed, So and Chan[13] found the inability to sleep in critical care units as a primary concern of both patients and nurses and suggested the need to revisit current practices in the promotion of sleep. Stewart and colleagues[3] found sleep quality in the ICU to be poor and noted that because there is an association between recovery and sleep, finding ways to improve sleep quality is essential to good patient care. Holistic approaches as independent nursing actions are of particular interest to ICU nurses who seek to "put the patient in the best condition for nature to act upon him."[14(p75)]

## HOLISM, HEALTH CARE, AND OPTIMAL HEALING ENVIRONMENTS

According to the World Health Organization's global report on traditional and complementary medicine 2019,[15] most of the world's population is reliant on herbal medicine. Herbal medicine and other holistic approaches are commonly referred to as CAM, or complementary and alternative medicine. The National Center for Complementary and Integrative Health (NCCIH)[16] differentiates complementary as a practice used or integrated with conventional medicine, and the term alternative medicine meaning it is being used in place of conventional medicine. Complementary approaches can be classified as natural products (eg, herbs, vitamins, and probiotics), mind and body practices (eg, yoga, chiropractic manipulation, and relaxation techniques), and other (eg, homeopathy, Ayurvedic medicine, and naturopathy). Nurses practice holistically, which pairs well with the concept of integrated health, where holistic approaches are used along with medical practices. Using mind-body approaches in coordination with conventional ICU therapies opens an opportunity to provide patient-centered care in a high-stress environment.

The American Holistic Nurses Association defines holism as both integral and unitary.[5] The nurse is encouraged to think of the interrelationship between the bio-psycho-social-spiritual dimensions as a whole, rather than placing the importance of that person into parts. The whole also includes the environment, which fits well with the recommendation that nurses assess for sleep disruptors in the ICU environment and develop sleep-promoting protocols to improve the systems of care for their patients.[6] Holistic approaches are interventions that focus on creation of optimal healing environments, which may include internal, interpersonal, behavioral, and external factors.[10] Using this model, (**Fig. 1**) highlights how holistic modalities discussed in this article fit into nursing practice focused on the whole. Internal elements are healing intentions from within a person. These may include personal motivation, mindfulness, spirituality, and religion. Interpersonal elements include both individual and organizational relationships. Behavioral factors are healthy lifestyle choices that include both western and eastern care practices. The last element is external, which would be the environment, systems of care or, in our focus, the ICU. Development of holistic protocols that promote sleep in the ICU should be sustainable in terms of the work of clinicians, acknowledge diversity of the population served, and recognize where they intersect with the 4 components of an optimal healing environment (see **Fig. 1**).

## DISCUSSION ON COMPLEMENTARY APPROACHES TO SLEEP

In a recent Cochrane review,[17] nonpharmacologic interventions were reviewed to promote sleep in the ICU. Reviewing studies up to 2014, 30 trials showed a wide range of interventions including psychological, complementary, environmental, social, and modification of ICU equipment. The investigators theorized that the use of complementary therapies to improve comfort, anxiety, and stress, which improved sleep in some patient populations, may be harder to use on patients who are critically ill and unconscious. Indeed, the investigators found it difficult to pool findings and reach a

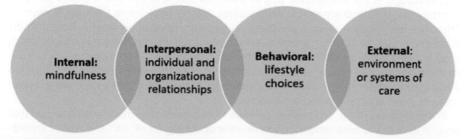

**Fig. 1.** Optimal Healing Environment framework. (*Adapted from* Sakallaris BR, MacAllister L, Voss M, et al. Optimal healing environments. Glob Adv Health Med. 2015;4(3):40; with permission.)

conclusion on effective interventions due to the variety of study designs and the lack of evidence quality. This conclusion was echoed in several reviews on integrative health, in which mind-body approaches augment and complement medical care.[9,17–20] Although these holistic approaches are favorable, they currently lack high levels of evidence for adoption as evidence-based interventions without further research.[8] One factor noted by researchers is that mind-body interventions may be harder to standardize and suggest the use of pilot studies to help define the "dosage" used to improve replication and comparison of outcomes in future studies.

As noted earlier, sleep is an intricate part of healing and has been noted as problematic by many researchers. In their review of the literature, DuBose and Hadi[21] discuss how the lack of quality sleep can lead to additional health concerns, which is why hospitals have tried different strategies to aid patients' sleep. Some modifiable environmental factors, such as noise and light, were themes in the 42 articles reviewed, but at the end of their review, they conclude that the research findings at that point in time were uneven and hard to consolidate. This was a function of many studies looking at multiple interventions. The investigators did conclude that there is great potential for using alternative approaches to improve sleep for hospital patients.

Hajibagheri and colleagues[22] also encourage us to seek complementary and alternative approaches to address patients' sleep, as many of the pharmacologic agents used in the ICU have untoward side effects. Patients in the ICU may be given benzodiazepines, opiates, or barbiturates as part of their medical care with the goal of easing pain and stress, and improving compliance with ventilation. These medications can affect REM activity and modify the circadian rhythm.[17] Given patients in the ICU already face serious health issues, reducing side effects while helping with sleep is seen as quite beneficial. Capezuti and colleagues[18] make the same recommendation, noting that some pharmacologic sleep aids can actually cause not only unwanted side effects, but increased falls for those patients who are mobile.

There are sufficient studies that recognize the need to improve sleep for hospitalized patients and the need to find effective alternative approaches for better sleep in the ICU setting.[6,8] In this article, we discuss the research on 3 holistic approaches to improve sleep for ICU patients. We believe these approaches show favorable effects on sleep and can be used as integrative practices to improve comfort in ICU patients, require minimal training to use, and are noninvasive. These approaches are part of the mind-body NCCIH classification, which we believe are easily implemented,[8] as well as show evidence of their efficacy for use in the ICU.

## AROMATHERAPY

Aromatherapy is the therapeutic use of essential oils. It is one of the oldest complementary and alternative medical approaches, dating back more than 6000 years.[23] There are numerous essential oils that can be used; ones often used in hospital settings are ginger, lavender, mandarin, and marjoram.[24] Aromatherapy is usually delivered in 1 of 3 ways: inhalation, through the skin, or orally.[23] In the research discussed in the following, we focus on aromatherapy studies that use inhalation to improve sleep quality. We consider this holistic approach to be part of the internal and external spheres in an optimal healing environment.

In the clinical setting, aromatherapy is used in a controlled manner with a goal that no one else in the area would notice an overwhelming smell with the use of aromatherapy. Clinical aromatherapy is not about masking odors in an environment; instead, it is used to trigger endocrine and immune system responses.[23] Buckle[25] notes that aromatherapy is often misunderstood and therefore underused. In fact, her review of pilot studies in the United States suggests that the integration of aromatherapy into patient care can have multiple positive outcomes, such as reduction in sleepiness and hospital-acquired infections like methicillin-resistant *Staphylococcus aureus* and vancomycin-resistant Enterococci.

Cho and colleagues[26] conducted a nonrandomized controlled trial to examine the effects of aromatherapy on ICU patients' stress and sleep quality. The study participants were patients admitted via the emergency room who spent more than 2 nights in the ICU. Importantly, for any patients with respiratory conditions, consent was obtained from a pulmonologist to use aromatherapy. The dosage of aromatherapy was determined by one of the researchers who was certified in the use of aromatherapy. Lavender was the essential oil used in this experiment. The Verran & Snyder-Halpern Sleep Scale (VSH) was used to measure sleep quality, which includes times waking up, tossing and turning, depth of sleep, how long to fall asleep, how one feels on waking up, and overall satisfaction with sleep. Higher scores indicated better sleep quality. For the control group, sleep quality decreased at each subsequent measure, from a mean of 61.03 at pretest to a mean of 25.80 at posttest2. For those who received the aromatherapy treatment, sleep quality also decreased, but to a statistically significantly lesser degree. It changed from a mean of 65.13 at pretest to a mean of 57.73 at posttest2. Sleep quality for the control group decreased by approximately 50%, whereas the drop for the treatment group was closer to 11%. Overall, the use of aromatherapy over 2 days increased the sleep quality of ICU patients.

Cho and colleagues[27] conducted a nonequivalent control group design to examine the effects of an aromatherapy blend (lavender, chamomile, and neroli) on patients in the ICU. There were 28 patients in the treatment group and 28 in the control group. Patients were asked to inhale the blended oils and also had aroma stones placed under their pillows during the night. They used the VSH, as translated into the Korean form. For this scale, higher scores indicate more satisfied sleep. Baseline measures were obtained on the day of admission and follow-up measures were taken after the percutaneous coronary intervention. Although both the treatment group and control group had similar VSH mean scores at baseline (53.0 and 55.6, respectively), after treatment, the treatment group had a mean score of 52.7, whereas the control group's mean dropped to 36.2, a difference significant at .001.

Şentürk and Tekinsoy Kartin[28] examined the use of lavender oil inhalation on the sleep quality of hemodialysis patients. They conducted a randomized controlled study, with 17 patients in the experimental group and 17 patients in the controlled group. The experimental group inhaled lavender oil every day for a week, whereas the controlled group had no exposure to the lavender oil. They used the PSQI to measure sleep quality, in which a score of less than 5 indicates good sleep quality and a score of 5 or higher indicates poor sleep quality. They also used the Daytime Sleepiness Level (DSL), measured as a visual analog scale, from 0 to 10, in which 0 represents a good sleep level. The results showed significant differences in the experimental group. Their DSL scores decreased from a mean of 6 to a mean of 3.82, whereas the change in the control group was from 5.76 to 5.52 (not significant). They also found significant differences in average sleeping times.

A simple, low-cost technique was used by Karadag and colleagues,[29] who examined the effects of aromatherapy on sleep quality of patients in the coronary ICU. As Karadag and colleagues[29] note, sleep quality has been found to be inversely related to the duration of stays in ICUs. Using a randomized controlled trial, lavender oil was inhaled by patients using a simple technique of 2 drops of oil on a piece of 2 × 2 gauze. Participants in the treatment group had the lavender-infused gauze pinned to their gown approximately 12 inches below the nose. This group was instructed to breathe normally and after 20 minutes the gauze was removed. The intervention took place before bedtime for a period of 15 days. The PSQI was used to measure sleep quality. For the treatment group, there was a statistically significant change toward better quality of sleep after 15 days of aromatherapy and there was no significant change in the control group.

Hajibagheri and colleagues[22] conducted a randomized controlled trial with Rosa damascene as the essential oil. They also used the PSQI to measure sleep quality. In this study, 3 drops of the essential oil was applied to a paper towel and attached to the side of the patient's pillow for 8 hours (22:00–06:00). This was done for 3 consecutive nights. For the total PSQI score, as well as 4 of the 6 subdomains, the treatment group had significantly better sleep quality than did the control group.

Simple aromatherapy techniques of using readily available materials, such as 2 × 2 gauze or paper towel mentioned previously can have positive effects on sleep quality. In a recent study, Johnson and colleagues[24] examined the use of several oils used for aromatherapy in an acute care setting. Although their focus was not on sleep, they outline the specific use of certain oils for pain, anxiety, and nausea, which can be linked to sleep difficulties. This was a retrospective study and included 7183 patients in which the specific aromatherapy essential oil was defined, and 3079 patients for whom the specific essential oil was not defined. Information on the identified symptom was recorded both before the use of aromatherapy and within 60 minutes of use. All 4 essential oils (ginger, lavender, mandarin, and sweet marjoram) were found to significantly reduce stress levels. Although more studies are needed, aromatherapy, using simple techniques is available for ICU nurses to consider as integrative practices and should be considered as part of the protocol developed to improve sleep in the ICU.

## GUIDED IMAGERY

Imagery techniques use the brain's natural image-making ability to influence physiology.[30] Most guided imagery relies on scripted material that can be read or recorded and is readily available for nurses to use for integrative practice.[30(p.282–289)] Another example can be found at Guided Imagery: https://www.guidedimageryinc.com/. The clinical effects from imagery techniques on physiology are well documented and include changes in heart rate, blood pressure, blood flow, pain, and immunity,[30,31] which may also improve sleep. According to Eliopoulos,[23] guided imagery is using one's imagination to create mental images that might relieve symptoms, promote relaxation, or otherwise help achieve a sense of well-being. A patient can use guided imagery alone or be led by a health care provider.

Loft and Cameron[32] conducted a 2 × 2 × 2 randomized controlled trial with New Zealand daytime workers across 10 companies with self-identified sleep disturbances. In this study, 104 participants were randomly assigned to 1 of 4 groups (control, arousal reduction, implementation intentions, and arousal reduction/ implementation intentions) to test the efficacy of those behavior interventions on sleep. These interventions were based on self-regulation therapy and all groups received laminated, written instructions, as well as audiotaped recordings of the instructions. Participants were contacted daily via e-mail and performed their instructed intervention twice daily (at the end of work and before going to bed). Pre-intervention data confirmed groups were similar. The study conclusions suggest imagery techniques positively affect sleep-related behavior in this small sample of daytime workers. The effects were statistically significant for sleep quality, time to sleep, and waking during sleep. The investigators did note the possibility that the focus on the issue of sleep through study participation may have had an effect on study results.

An older narrative review identified that relaxation and guided imagery are significantly associated with improvements in sleep quality, vital signs, pain quality, complications, length of stay, and patient satisfaction.[33] Of the 14 studies reviewed, all interventions took place at a single site using convenience sampling, and most participants had a cardiovascular-related diagnosis, so generalizability may be limited. Even with these limitations, the participants viewed the supportive nurse-patient interaction or psychosocial interventions as helpful to extremely helpful. The investigators selected studies where psychological/emotional support, relaxation, and imagery interventions were used. Guided imagery was "defined as a way of purposefully diverting and focusing one's thoughts."[33(p120)] The study concluded that the amount of nurse attention needed to perform these psychological support interventions may be a factor, but that these interventions had a positive effect on ICU patients, nonetheless. In addition, this study identified the scarcity of studies exploring nurse-mediated support interventions between 1970 and 2010.

A high degree of sleep disturbance in the ICU prompted a repeated measures experimental study to gauge the effects of relaxation and guided imagery on sleep.[34] Thirty-six adult ICU patients who agreed to participate were randomly placed in 1 of 2 groups, experimental or control. Over a 3-day period, both groups participated in initial data collection on day 1, and measures of sleep quality on days 2 and 3. The experimental group experienced 1 relaxation session using scripted 1:1 in-person delivery and guided imagery using patient-selected images. The data collected did not support the initial hypothesis that sleep scores would increase over time in the experimental group; however, the investigators found female patients may respond better to this type of intervention, and transfer out of the ICU improved scores.

Variability in patient outcomes post coronary artery bypass graft (CABG) surgery triggered a replication study to use guided imagery to improve anxiety, pain, narcotic use, fatigue, patient satisfaction, and length of stay.[34,35] Using the theoretic framework from the Center for Advanced Practice Evidence-based Practice Model, researchers recruited 100 patients, split evenly into control and intervention groups, which were well matched for comparison. The intervention is well documented and included 2 prerecorded tapes developed and used in a previous study.[36] Outcome measures were lower in the intervention group, although very few were significantly lower, suggesting the use of the intervention protocol, which is simple and low-cost, may have a positive effect on persons undergoing CABG surgery.

Spiva and colleagues focused on the effects of guided imagery on mechanically ventilated patients. Although outcome variables were not specifically associated with sleep, pain control and sedation are recognized as factors that affect sleep quality. Two hospitals within an integrated health system were used to recruit patients from 7 different ICUs into an intervention and control group over an 18-month period. One hospital served as the control group, having similar patient populations to the hospital using the intervention. The intervention took place during 2 morning weaning trials using prerecorded 60-minute guided imagery audio sessions with the researcher present. The Richmond Agitation-Sedation Scale (RASS) was used to measure sedation and pain control, illness severity was measured using the Acute Physiology and Chronic Health Evaluation (APACHE II), and researchers developed their own scale to measure feasibility and satisfaction using guided imagery by nurses. Comparison groups were slightly different, most notably in gender, race, and a tendency for the intervention group to have higher RASS scores and to be maintained on continuous sedation. APACHE scores were similar (control M = 22.9; intervention M = 25.8). Given the intervention group may have been sicker and needing more sedation, it is both statistically and clinically significant that their RASS scores improved with guided imagery, as well as decreasing their time on the ventilator. The investigators felt guided imagery had a positive effect and should be part of the multimodal treatment plan for ventilator weaning.

Guided imagery scripts are readily available to adopt and should be considered for integrative practice in protocol development to improve sleep quality in the ICU. This method is an independent nursing action that can be easily used and has shown positive effects on sleep quality. Although some studies indicated the intervention effect may have been related to the supportive nurse-patient interaction or psychosocial intervention, not the guided imagery itself, it still provides a patient-centered positive effect. In the Optimal Healing Environment this holistic approach is focused on interpersonal relationships.

## MINDFULNESS-BASED INTERVENTIONS

In this section, we focus on mindfulness-based interventions (MBI), which are a form of meditation, and are a holistic approach focused on the internal sphere of the healing environment. It is important to distinguish MBI from meditation, as meditation usually requires a lengthy period of learning and practice before one can become adept at the practice.[37] Mindfulness, on the other hand, is a practice that can be done with little or no training, and can be facilitated through the use of smartphone applications. A Mayo Clinic[38] article discusses how forms of meditation can be simple and even fast ways to reduce stress. Furthermore, related to illness, the article notes that sleep problems are one thing that can be improved with mindfulness practices. Nunez[39] discusses 3 ways that meditation can improve sleep, with one way being simple breathing practices.

As with guided imagery, MBIs are a form of mind-body therapies that focus on the relationships of the mind, body, and brain. Similar to meditation, these interventions are designed to focus attention on what is going on in the present, most notably as a way to help the entire system reach a relaxed state.[23] Mindfulness helps a person to focus on what is going on in the immediate moment, which usually involves letting go of thoughts that may distract from the present time, promoting a healthy internal health environment. The use of mindfulness has been shown to reduce anxiety and depression, both of which can impact the quality of sleep. In addition, "[mindfulness] has been shown to decrease ruminative thoughts, diminish emotional reactivity, and promote reappraisal of salient experiences, which together may facilitate sleep."[19(p2)] The ICU is a perfect example of a time when we cannot change the environment or the source of stress.[40] This is where mindfulness-based practices can be helpful, as they promote changing the relationship a person has with stress. In their review of literature between 2008 and 2019, Ong and Moore[40] found evidence that MBIs are strongest at reducing total wake time, even though the effect on total sleep time was not statistically significant. Therefore, using mindfulness-based practices might help patients relax more and be less stressed, 2 qualities that can impact sleep.

Mindfulness practices, especially as might be implemented in the ICU, are not the same as mindfulness-based stress reduction (MBSR) practices, which usually require an 8-week training program. We highlight a few findings on MBSR as a way to note findings related to mindfulness-based practices and then more directly discuss mindfulness practices that are not a part of MBSR. In addition, although MBSR may not be practical in the ICU setting, MBSR practices may be useful in the weeks and months post-ICU when patients are recovering. An introduction to mindfulness practices in the ICU may trigger changes in behavior and lifestyle, enhancing that optimal healing environment in this recovery stage.

Ong and Moore[40] conducted a systematic review of research on mindfulness and sleep. First they presented their metacognitive model on why mindfulness might relate to sleep. As they note, "Sleep disturbance most commonly occurs when there is dysregulation in these systems accompanied by activation of the sympathetic nervous system, creating a state of hyperarousal."[40(p18)] These systems are the systems of the body that govern homeostatic pressure and circadian rhythms. They found that, in general, MBIs can improve sleep quality. In 2 studies of mindfulness-based meditation, findings showed that the use of mindfulness-based meditation can result in statistically significant changes in sleep quality.[40,41] In the study by Black and colleagues,[41] the treatment group learned mindfulness-based meditation while the control group learned sleep hygiene. The treatment group had significant improvement in sleep quality, as measured by the PSQI. For Gross and colleagues,[42] subjects with insomnia were placed into the MBSR treatment group while the control group was provided pharmacotherapy. Gross and colleagues[42] used several measures for sleep quality, including measures of insomnia (Insomnia Sleep Index), the PSQI, the Dysfunctional Beliefs and Attitudes about Sleep, and Sleep Self-Efficacy Scale. Overall, Gross and colleagues[42] found that the use of MBSR, along with information on sleep hygiene, had a significant impact on sleep quality. They found a similar impact with the use of pharmacotherapy, suggesting mindfulness-based meditation would be an acceptable substitute for the use of drugs.

Systematic reviews have been conducted on the use of mindfulness-based meditation and sleep quality. For Rusch and colleagues,[19] their search and inclusion/exclusion criteria resulted in 79 articles, ranging in date from 2010 to 2018. They found moderate strength of evidence for MBIs improving sleep quality compared with control groups, both at postintervention and at follow-up. In their systematic review of the literature, Winbush and colleagues[20] examined 7 articles that met their search criteria. Of those, 4 reported significantly improved sleep quality for those who used MBSR. None of these 4 studies used a control group, and the other 3 studies did not find a significant difference between MBSR and the control group. They conclude that the available evidence suggests the need for better-designed trials to fully examine the effects of MBSR on sleep, both quality and duration. Specifically, there is a need for randomized and controlled study designs and greater adherence to standardized measures of mindfulness-based meditation.

Jain and colleagues[43] conducted a randomized controlled trial examining the effects of mindfulness meditation versus relaxation training in health care students. They found significant effects for both the mindfulness and relaxation groups, noting that the effect size for the mindfulness group was considerably larger than that of the relaxation group (0.71 and 0.25, respectively). In a meta-analysis of mindfulness meditation for insomnia, researchers found that compared with the control group, mindfulness meditation significantly reduced total wake time, sleep-onset latency, and scores on the PSQI, and increased both sleep quality and efficiency.[44]

Unfortunately, most of the empirical work on mindfulness is specific to mindfulness meditation, especially MBSR, as first articulated by Kabat-Zinn.[45] Although MBSR has been shown to be effective at increasing sleep quality and improving other aspects of health and well-being, it may not be suited to work in the ICU, as it requires too lengthy a time for training. What may work in the ICU are quick techniques to introduce people to mindfulness practices. Mindfulness practices can help improve sleep by addressing what might be happening in the sympathetic nervous system. Sood and Jones[46] examined various mindfulness practices by measuring their impact through MRI scans. They looked at both focused attention and open wandering techniques. Focused attention is well aligned with mindfulness practices we discuss, as it allows attention to one sensory experience, such as the breath. A goal of focused attention is to shift the person's focus from self-preoccupation or mind wandering to the present moment. They found that such mindfulness practices can lead to increased relaxation, which, in turn, decreases activity of the sympathetic nervous system. A stimulated sympathetic nervous system can lead to a state of hyperarousal, which impedes the ability to go to sleep.

Three practices (use of smartphone-based applications, S.TO.P. [described later in this article], and mindfulness-based breathing/attention activities) are described to consider for use in the ICU to improve relaxation and improve sleep. Key to what we review are practices that can help the ICU patient to either move their attention from an inability to sleep to an awareness of what might be getting in the way of their sleep or transcend (accept) their circumstances such that they can shift into a greater ability to fall asleep.

Mindfulness applications on a smartphone show promising applicability to the ICU setting. As opposed to MBSRs that are time and cost intensive, mobile technologies may prove convenient and easy to use once people are aware of their availability. Rung and colleagues[47] invited 2852 WaTCH participants to use a mobile mindfulness app (Headspace) for at least 10 of the following 30 days. Self-report surveys were used to measure feasibility, participation, retention, and acceptability of the app in the 236 participants of 318 who completed the follow-up survey. Health-related outcomes were focused on trait mindfulness, depressive symptoms, perceived stress, sleep quality, physical activity, body mass index, and healthy eating. Of particular interest to this review is sleep quality, which most of these participants reported as being improved in 3 areas of the PSQI, measuring self-reported sleep quality, sleep duration, and sleep latency.

S.T.O.P., developed by Stahl and Goldstein,[48] is a simple practice in which the person, finding themselves unable to sleep, takes a few minutes to check in with what might be happening. First you Stop what you are doing, Take a breath, Observe what is going on around you, and Proceed. The ICU nurse is well positioned to use this type of mindfulness technique to assist the patient. Taking only a few moments, this might help the patient focus on a sound that is disturbing them or something else within the ICU setting that can be modified to improve comfort. As Reuter-Rice and colleagues[6] identified, there are environmental factors (eg, light, intrusive monitoring, and interventions) that may be modified to improve the sleeping environment. Using S.T.O.P. is a patient-centered technique that takes just minutes to use, and the patient now has the awareness to ask the clinical staff for help, such as ear plugs, an eye cover, or something else.

Mindfulness-based breathing exercises are a ready tool for anyone, and often serve as the foundation for meditation practices. The breath is always with you, no matter where you are and can be used as a tool to bring your focus to the present moment.[48] Although abdominal breathing is often recommended, it is not required, as it is important for the practice that the person breathe in a way that works for them. Mindful breathing can be done sitting up or lying down, which makes it easily accessible for patients in the ICU. Techniques developed by Stahl and Goldstein[48] are well suited to use in the ICU, as the technique could be as simple as 5 minutes of mindful breathing. Stahl and Goldstein[48] provide scripts for each mindful breathing practice and the script could be presented digitally to the patient, a nurse could read the script, the patient could read the script, or download it here: https://elishagoldstein.com/ecourses/basics-of-mindfulness-meditation/resources/

Golfenshtein and colleagues[49] did a qualitative study of mothers whose infants were in the cardiac ICU. Using purposive sampling, they recruited 14 women to participate in the study. All of the mothers noted high levels of stress and reported both active and passive ways of coping with such stress. The mothers were provided an overview of a mindfulness practice, asked how they thought it might help them with their stress, participated in a 10-minute self-practice session, and were then interviewed on their experiences. The researchers note that most of the mothers "expressed overall positive reactions following the breathing demo session, reporting on increased focusing abilities. They especially favored the simplicity, accessibility, and versatility of the practice."[49(p123)] Although not a randomized controlled trial, this study does suggest that simple mindfulness breathing practices can reduce stress and help participants better cope with their situation. Lessened stress can be directly linked to improved sleep.

There are several limitations to the research, a primary one being how to measure mindfulness,[44] as there are accepted measures of sleep quality, such as the PSQI, the Insomnia Sleep Index, and the Medical Outcomes Study-Sleep Scale. As noted previously, mindfulness as used in this article is not the same as mindfulness meditation or MBSR, as the latter often requires training that far exceeds time in the ICU. However, defining mindfulness as short and accessible breathing practices would allow us to better explore how mindfulness might help with sleep in the ICU.

Another limitation is raised by Ong and Moore,[40] who note that using mindfulness to achieve sleep is antithetical to a key meditation principle, which is nonattachment to outcome.[39] However, for the short breathing practices we discuss, outcome is an included factor, unlike the more elaborate meditation practices. Other limitations, as noted previously, include lack of consistent measures of both sleep quality and mindfulness techniques. Even when there is agreement on how to measure sleep, studies need to take into consideration whether there are comorbid conditions that could impact sleep quality.[40] Overall, however, research does indicate positive impacts of MBIs on sleep, suggesting mindfulness-based techniques could be helpful to ICU patients.

## SUMMARY

ICU patients experience internal, interpersonal, behavioral, and environmental factors that can disrupt their sleep. The major focus of altering these disruptions in the research has been on modifying environmental factors such as noise, lighting practices, patient care activities, diagnostic procedures, and the use of sedatives and analgesics.[2,5,6] It has been suggested that additional sleep promotion protocols be developed to improve sleep quality in ICU units, although this is not yet common.[6] Sleep protocols that are holistic will include factors that address all spheres of the Optimal Healing Environment (internal, interpersonal, behavioral, and environmental),[10] are cost-effective, easy to use, and independent nursing actions that are integrative in nature. It is acknowledged that patients who are critically ill and unconscious or mechanically ventilated pose some challenge to holistic approaches that require patient participation. For that reason, aromatherapy, guided imagery, and mindfulness were chosen for their ease of use and promising effect to improve comfort, anxiety, and stress, which improved sleep in some patient populations.

## CLINICS CARE POINTS

- Holistic practices promote an optimal healing environment.
- ICU patients can have better sleep.

- Variety of protocols allows for better patient-centered care.
- Key is integration, across the environment and care team.
- Focus should be on clinical approaches to use.
- Be attentive to patient preferences.

## DISCLOSURE

The authors have nothing to disclose.

## REFERENCES

1. Sheehan CM, Frochen SE, Walsemann KM, et al. Are U.S. adults reporting less sleep? Findings from sleep duration trends in the National Health Interview Survey, 2004–2017. Sleep 2019;(2):42. https://doi.org/10.1093/sleep/zsy221.
2. Pisani MA, Friese RS, Gehlbach BK, et al. Sleep in the intensive care unit. Am J Respir Crit Care Med 2015;191(7):731–8.
3. Stewart JA, Green C, Stewart J, et al. Factors influencing quality of sleep among non-mechanically ventilated patients in the Intensive Care Unit. Aust Crit Care 2017;30(2):85–90.
4. Devlin JW, Skrobik Y, Gélinas C, et al. Clinical Practice Guidelines for the prevention and management of pain, agitation/sedation, delirium, immobility, and sleep disruption in adult patients in the ICU. Crit Care Med 2018;46(9):e825.
5. Dossey BM, Keegan L, Barrere C, et al, editors. Holistic nursing: a handbook for practice. 7th edition. Burlington, MA: Jones & Bartlett Learning; 2016.
6. Reuter-Rice K, McMurray MG, Christoferson E, et al. Sleep in the intensive care unit. Crit Care Nurs Clin North Am 2020;32(2):191–201.
7. Kolcaba K. Comfort theory and practice: a vision for holistic health care and research. New York: Springer Pub. Co; 2003.
8. Papathanassoglou E, Park T. To put the patient in the best condition: integrating integrative therapies in critical care. Nurs Crit Care 2016;21(3):123–6.
9. Altman MT, Knauert MP, Pisani MA. Sleep disturbance after hospitalization and critical illness: a systematic review. Ann Am Thorac Soc 2017;14(9):1457–68.
10. Sakallaris BR, MacAllister L, Voss M, et al. Optimal healing environments. Glob Adv Health Med 2015;4(3):40–5.
11. Buysse DJ, Reynolds CF, Monk TH, et al. The Pittsburgh Sleep Quality Index: a new instrument for psychiatric practice and research. Psychiatry Res 1989; 28(2):193–213.
12. Maslow AH. Classics in the history of psychology – A. H. Maslow (1943), a theory of human motivation. Available at: https://psychclassics.yorku.ca/Maslow/motivation.htm. Accessed October 29, 2020.
13. So HM, Chan DSK. Perception of stressors by patients and nurses of critical care units in Hong Kong. Int J Nurs Stud 2004;41(1):77–84.
14. Nightingale F. Notes on nursing 1860. Available at: https://digital.library.upenn.edu/women/nightingale/nursing/nursing.html. Accessed October 29, 2020.
15. World Health Organization, editor. WHO global report on traditional and complementary medicine, 2019. Geneva, Switzerland: World Health Organization; 2019.
16. The National Center for Complementary and Integrative Health. Complementary, alternative, or integrative health: what's in a Name? NCCIH. Available at: https://

www.nccih.nih.gov/health/complementary-alternative-or-integrative-health-whats-in-a-name. Accessed October 29, 2020.

17. Hu R-F, Jiang X-Y, Chen J, et al. Non-pharmacological interventions for sleep promotion in the intensive care unit. Cochrane Database Syst Rev 2015;10. https://doi.org/10.1002/14651858.CD008808.pub2.

18. Capezuti E, Sagha Zadeh R, Pain K, et al. A systematic review of non-pharmacological interventions to improve nighttime sleep among residents of long-term care settings. BMC Geriatr 2018;18(1):143.

19. Rusch HL, Rosario M, Levison LM, et al. The effect of mindfulness meditation on sleep quality: a systematic review and meta-analysis of randomized controlled trials. Ann N Y Acad Sci 2019;1445(1):5–16.

20. Winbush NY, Gross CR, Kreitzer MJ. The effects of mindfulness-based stress reduction on sleep disturbance: a systematic review. Explore (NY) 2007;3(6):585–91.

21. DuBose JR, Hadi K. Improving inpatient environments to support patient sleep. Int J Qual Health Care 2016;28(5):540–53.

22. Hajibagheri A, Babaii A, Adib-Hajbaghery M. Effect of rosa damascene aromatherapy on sleep quality in cardiac patients: a randomized controlled trial. Complement Ther Clin Pract 2014;20(3):159–63.

23. Eliopoulos C. Invitation to holistic health: a guide to living a balanced life. 4th edition. Burlington, MA: Jones & Bartlett Learning; 2018.

24. Johnson JR, Rivard RL, Griffin KH, et al. The effectiveness of nurse-delivered aromatherapy in an acute care setting. Complement Ther Med 2016;25:164–9.

25. Buckle J. Literature review: should nursing take aromatherapy more seriously? Br J Nurs 2007;16(2):116–20.

26. Cho EH, Lee M-Y, Hur M-H. The effects of aromatherapy on intensive care unit patients' stress and sleep quality: a nonrandomised controlled trial. Evid Based Complement Alternat Med 2017;2017:2856592.

27. Cho M-Y, Min ES, Hur M-H, et al. Effects of aromatherapy on the anxiety, vital signs, and sleep quality of percutaneous coronary intervention patients in intensive care units. Evid Based Complement Alternat Med 2013;2013:381381.

28. Şentürk A, Tekinsoy Kartın P. The effect of lavender oil application via inhalation pathway on hemodialysis patients' anxiety level and sleep quality. Holist Nurs Pract 2018;32(6):324–35.

29. Karadag E, Samancioglu S, Ozden D, et al. Effects of aromatherapy on sleep quality and anxiety of patients. Nurs Crit Care 2017;22(2):105–12.

30. Schaub B, Burt M. Imagery. In: Dossey B, Keegan L, editors. Holistic nursing. A handbook for practice. 7th edition. Burlington, MA: Jones & Bartlett Learning; 2016. p. 282–9.

31. Sheikh AA. Healing images: the role of imagination in health. 1st edition. Amityville, NY: Routledge; 2002.

32. Loft MH, Cameron LD. Using mental imagery to deliver self-regulation techniques to improve sleep behaviors. Ann Behav Med 2013;46(3):260–72.

33. Papathanassoglou EDE. Psychological support and outcomes for ICU patients. Nurs Crit Care 2010;15(3):118–28.

34. Richardson S. Effects of relaxation and imagery on the sleep of critically ill adults. Dimens Crit Care Nurs 2003;22(4):182–90.

35. Deisch P, Soukup SM, Adams P, et al. Guided imagery: replication study using coronary artery bypass graft patients. Nurs Clin North Am 2000;35(2):417–25.

36. Tusek D, Church JM, Fazio VW. Guided imagery as a coping strategy for perioperative patients. AORN J 1997;66(4):644–9.

37. Goyal M, Singh S, Sibinga EMS, et al. Meditation programs for psychological stress and well-being: A systematic review and meta-analysis. JAMA Intern Med 2014;174(3):357–68.
38. Mayo Clinic. A beginner's guide to meditation. Mayo Clinic. Available at: https://www.mayoclinic.org/tests-procedures/meditation/in-depth/meditation/art-20045858. Accessed October 29, 2020.
39. Nunez K. Meditation for Sleep: How to Use Meditation for Insomnia, Better Sleep. Healthline. Published January 13, 2020. Available at: https://www.healthline.com/health/meditation-for-sleep. Accessed October 29, 2020.
40. Ong JC, Moore C. What do we really know about mindfulness and sleep health? Curr Opin Psychol 2020;34:18–22.
41. Black DS, O'Reilly GA, Olmstead R, et al. Mindfulness meditation and improvement in sleep quality and daytime impairment among older adults with sleep disturbances. JAMA Intern Med 2015;175(4):494–501.
42. Gross CR, Kreitzer MJ, Reilly-Spong M, et al. Mindfulness-based stress reduction versus pharmacotherapy for chronic primary insomnia: a randomized controlled clinical trial. Explore (NY) 2011;7(2):76–87.
43. Jain S, Shapiro SL, Swanick S, et al. A randomized controlled trial of mindfulness meditation versus relaxation training: effects on distress, positive states of mind, rumination, and distraction. Ann Behav Med 2007;33(1):11–21.
44. Gong H, Ni C-X, Liu Y-Z, et al. Mindfulness meditation for insomnia: a meta-analysis of randomized controlled trials. J Psychosom Res 2016;89:1–6.
45. Kabat-Zinn J. Full catastrophe living: using the wisdom of your body and mind to face stress, pain, and illness. New York: Bantam Books; 1990.
46. Sood A, Jones DT. On mind wandering, attention, brain networks, and meditation. Explore 2013;9(3):136–41.
47. Rung AL, Oral E, Berghammer L, et al. Feasibility and acceptability of a mobile mindfulness meditation intervention among women: intervention study. JMIR Mhealth Uhealth 2020;8(6):e15943.
48. Stahl B, Goldstein E. A mindfulness-based stress reduction workbook. Oakland, CA: New Harbinger Publications; 2010.
49. Golfenshtein N, Deatrick JA, Lisanti AJ, et al. Coping with stress in the cardiac intensive care unit: can mindfulness be the answer? J Pediatr Nurs 2017;37: 117–26.

# Review of Pharmacologic Sleep Agents for Critically Ill Patients

Kaylee Marino, PharmD, BCCCP, BCPS,
Melanie Goodberlet, PharmD, BCCCP, BCPS*,
Patricia Cyrus, PharmD, BCPS

## KEYWORDS

- Sleep • Insomnia • Pharmacology • Medications • Critical care

## KEY POINTS

- Sleep disruption is common in critically ill patients. Sleep disruption may become compromised and difficult to detect in this patient population.
- The use of some sedative pharmacologic agents may continue to interfere with deep restorative sleep. It is important to be cognizant of the mechanism of sleep promotion for these agents.
- Optimization of sleep in critically ill patients should include nonpharmacologic and pharmacologic means that are tailored to patient- and disease-specific factors.

## BACKGROUND

Sleep is a dynamic process that aids in mental and physical restoration.[1] Normal sleep is divided into non-REM (NREM) and REM sleep. NREM is divided into 4 stages and progresses into deep sleep.[2] REM sleep resembles wakefulness on an electroencephalogram; however, muscle activity is diminished—it is considered to be restful sleep and is associated with dreaming.[2] REM sleep is also categorized by variable levels of sympathetic and parasympathetic stimulation and the arousal threshold.[2] Sudden increases in sympathetic activity correlate with changes in blood pressure, heart rate, and respiratory rate.[2] Sleep disruption can be categorized into several subgroups but overarchingly refers to changes in sleep quantity, quality, or interruption of the circadian rhythm.[3]

It is reported that 46% to 100% of patients admitted to intensive care units (ICU) have inadequate sleep secondary to critical illness, procedures and interventions, medications, and monitoring.[1] It is important to note that although a patient may be asleep or sedated, their sleep architecture can still be compromised. Friese[4] discovered that sleep architecture in the ICU was mostly composed of light sleep (NREM stages 1 and 2) with

Department of Pharmacy, Brigham and Women's Hospital, 75 Francis Street, Boston, MA 02215, USA
* Corresponding author.
E-mail address: mgoodberlet@partners.org

Crit Care Nurs Clin N Am 33 (2021) 145–153
https://doi.org/10.1016/j.cnc.2021.01.006
0899-5885/21/Published by Elsevier Inc.

very little time spent in the deeper and more restorative stages. Interestingly, the use of opioids in escalating doses has been shown to increase wakefulness and stage 2 NREM sleep through stimulation of the pontothalamic pathway.[2] However, if pain is inhibiting sleep, the use of opioids may promote sleep through this indirect analgesic mechanism. The effect of other commonly used sedatives on the sleep architecture will be discussed throughout the review. Inadequate sleep in this population increases the risk of delirium, cognitive and immune system dysfunction, altered metabolism, prolonged mechanical ventilation, and psychological distress.[1,2,5,6] Sleep impairment itself has been identified as a stressor and may additionally hinder a fast and successful recovery.[7]

In 2020, Honarmand and colleagues[3] conducted a systematic review of 62 studies in an attempt to better identify risk factors for sleep disruption in critically ill patients; the most commonly reported factors by patients included pain, discomfort, anxiety and fear, noise, light, and ICU care-related activities. Of these factors, noise and light were rated by patients as the most disruptive factors.[3] As summarized in this review and in other studies, nonpharmacologic therapy and the minimization of nocturnal stimuli are effective in promoting sleep and preserving circadian rhythm. However, many patients require additional pharmacologic aid.[1,5] The objective of this article is to summarize the different options and usefulness of available therapies for sleep disturbances in the ICU.

## NONPHARMACOLOGIC MANAGEMENT

Interventions for sleep promotion include pharmacologic and nonpharmacologic options. The 2018 Clinical Practice Guidelines for the Prevention and Management of Pain, Agitation/Sedation, Delirium, Immobility, and Sleep Disruption in Adult Patients in the ICU (PADIS) recommend noise and light reduction strategies to improve sleep in critically ill adults.[8] Two studies compared the use of ear plugs and eye masks versus usual care and assessed nurse-measured sleep quantity. These studies found that total sleep time was significantly greater in the intervention group compared with the control group. Additionally, patients in the ear plugs and eye masks group displayed less mild confusion and delirium.[9,10] Despite these 2 studies, the overall quality of evidence remains low for the use of earplugs or masks. Additional noise reduction strategies include individual rooms, closing doors to patient rooms, lowering alarm volume levels when able on medical equipment such as ventilators and dialysis machines, customized monitors, and other equipment based on each patient's illness, and minimizing conversations at or near the patient's bedside during the evening and overnight hours.[4] Light reduction strategies include promotion of natural light during the day to start and support the circadian rhythm, and minimizing or dimming lights at night time.[4,11] Although the promotion and maintenance of sleep is important in critically ill patients, it is recognized that routine ICU care should not be withheld if necessary to implement during the evening (ie, neurologic assessment after administration of alteplase).

## MELATONIN AND RAMELTEON

Physiologic melatonin is secreted at night and synchronizes the sleep/wake and dark/light cycles.[2] It plays an integral role in circadian rhythm and reduction in plasma levels have been seen in critically ill patients on mechanical ventilation.[12] Most commonly used doses range from 3 to 10 mg (mg) and should be administered 30 to 60 minutes before bedtime.[13] Melatonin has few mild adverse effects (ie, mild sedation, headache) even at extremely high doses.[12] Dependence and tolerance have not been reported. These factors, in combination with its low cost, have made melatonin an attractive option for sleep promotion.

Because melatonin manufacturing is not regulated by the US Food and Drug Administration (FDA), concerns have been raised regarding quality and consistency. In an effort to address this concern, ramelteon (a melatonin 1 and 2 receptor agonist) was created. If used, ramelteon is dosed as 8 mg nightly administered 30 minutes before sleep.[14] Similarly to melatonin, it is well-tolerated with few adverse effects; however, it does carry a higher cost when compared with melatonin.[15] Ramelteon should not be used with CYP1A2 enzyme inhibitors owing to elevated levels of ramelteon.[14]

The current literature evaluating the use of melatonin and ramelteon have yielded mixed results.[12,16,17] Some studies reported a small improvement in sleep quality, but the evidence is not strong enough for expert guidelines to make a recommendation. The current studies also cite a potential improvement in sleep latency; however, there has been no demonstrated effect on total sleep time, sleep fragmentation, or sleep efficiency.[18] The PADIS guidelines do not make a recommendation regarding the use of melatonin or ramelteon in critically ill adults.[8]

## PROPOFOL

Propofol is a sedative that is approved by the FDA for general anesthesia, sedation of mechanically ventilated patients, and procedural sedation. It exerts its sedative action through activation of the gamma-aminobutyric acid A (GABA-A) receptor, the primary inhibitory neurotransmitter in the central nervous system.[19] It has a rapid onset of action (30–45 seconds) as well as recovery.[19] Although propofol has been studied for the promotion of sleep in critically ill patients, there has been no demonstratable improvement in sleep when compared with placebo.[20] Additionally, suppression of stage 4 and REM sleep and worsened sleep quality have been observed in clinical trials.[2,21] There also is significant potential for hypotension, bradycardia, and respiratory depression. Propofol is not recommended by the PADIS guidelines for the purpose of improving sleep in critically ill patients.[8]

## DEXMEDETOMIDINE

Dexmedetomidine is a selective central alpha-2 adrenergic receptor agonist used for sedation in the ICU and procedural settings. It exhibits sedative, anxiolytic, and analgesic properties with minimal respiratory depression.[22] Two randomized trials have compared dexmedetomidine with placebo for sleep in critically ill mechanically ventilated patients and in critically ill non–mechanically ventilated patients not requiring a continuous sedative infusion. Dexmedetomidine increased stage 2 sleep and decreased stage 1 sleep in both studies. However, the studies did not show a decrease in sleep fragmentation or an increase in deep or REM sleep.[23,24] Another study has shown preserved day–night cycling when dexmedetomidine was administered overnight in mechanically ventilated critical care patients.[25] Despite minimal respiratory depression, dexmedetomidine does have peripheral effects, including bradycardia and vasodilation resulting in hypotension, so close hemodynamic monitoring is required. Given the potential benefit on sleep architecture, the PADIS guidelines advise dexmedetomidine could be considered in hemodynamically stable critically ill patients who require a sedative infusion overnight.[8]

## BENZODIAZEPINES, BARBITURATES, AND HYPNOTICS

There are 5 benzodiazepines that are FDA approved for the treatment of insomnia: triazolam, estazolam, temazepam, quazepam, and flurazepam. Benzodiazepines are GABA receptor agonists that promote sleep, decrease anxiety, and provide muscle relaxation.[26] Although benzodiazepines are FDA approved for the treatment of insomnia, studies have demonstrated a potentially detrimental effect on sleep architecture. At low doses, benzodiazepines decrease deep and REM sleep, and increase stage 2 NREM sleep. With repeated use, stage 4 NREM sleep may be completely absent.[2] Additionally, they are not without adverse effects, addictive properties, tolerance, and withdrawal consequences if stopped abruptly. All of these agents are schedule IV controlled substances owing their potential for abuse and/or dependence.[27] Benzodiazepines should be avoided or used with extreme caution in elderly patients because of their increased sensitivity and slower metabolism of long-acting agents. Benzodiazepines can increase the risk of cognitive impairment, delirium, falls, and fractures in the elderly population.[28] Additionally, in the critical care setting, benzodiazepines are not recommended routinely for sedation management owing to side effects, an increased risk of delirium, and accumulation. Of note, the PADIS guidelines recommend propofol or dexmedetomidine over benzodiazepines for sedation in critically ill, mechanically ventilated adults for these reasons.[8] In the medical and surgical adult ICU patient population, a nonbenzodiazepine intravenous sedative regimen was associated with a shorter ICU length of stay and shorter duration of mechanical ventilation when compared with those patients receiving benzodiazepines for sedation. The study did not demonstrate a difference in mortality.[29]

The "Z drug" agents also work as GABA agonists on the GABA-A receptor and include zaleplon, zolpidem, and eszopiclone. These agents exert their effect for short-term insomnia by binding to the benzodiazepine site of the alpha-1 subunit of the GABA-A receptor complex, increasing the frequency of chloride channel opening and resulting in inhibition of neuronal excitation.[30–32] When compared with placebo, Z drugs produced a small, dose-dependent improvement in subjective and polysomographic sleep latency of 7 minutes and 22 minutes, respectively. The authors concluded that the clinical significance of such a small difference is uncertain and needs to be balanced with the adverse effects of this drug class.[33] Eszopiclone has the longest half-life (6 hours) compared with zolpidem (1–2 hours) and zaleplon (1 hour). In general, the onset of these medications is quicker if taken on an empty stomach, with zalepon having the quickest onset followed by zolpidem and eszopiclone.[30–32] Similar to benzodiazepines, these medications are known to cause tolerance and have abuse potential. Additional adverse effects include hallucinations and delusions.[33]

Barbiturates act by increasing the frequency and duration of opening the chloride ion channel in the GABA-A receptor complex through a different binding site than benzodiazepines.[26] Although effective for sleep, they also impair the length of time in deep and REM sleep, have a narrow therapeutic index, and produce a cross-tolerance to other GABA-A agonist sedating drugs, including alcohol and benzodiazepines.[2,26] Owing to the risk of cardiac and respiratory depression, addictive potential, drug interactions, and cognitive impairment, barbiturates are not recommended for the treatment of insomnia.

## ANTIDEPRESSANTS

Antidepressants may be used for the treatment of insomnia; however, this use is considered "off-label" owing to poor evidence and a lack of FDA approval for this indication. Despite this, many providers gravitate toward the use of antidepressants out of concern for the abuse and dependence potential associated with the hypnotic agents. All antidepressants suppress REM sleep except trazodone.[34] The sedating effects are primarily mediated via histamine and/or serotonin. Tolerance to the sedating effects (as well as anticholinergic effects) usually develop within 1 to 2 weeks, although the

REM suppressing effects can remain. A recent Cochrane review identified a small number of quality studies for the use of antidepressants for managing primary insomnia. The evidence provided only marginal data supporting short-term use for some tricyclic antidepressants (TCAs), mainly doxepin and trazodone.[35] Given the lack of supporting data and potential for adverse effects, the routine use of antidepressants (aside from low-dose doxepin) for insomnia is not recommended in patients who are not diagnosed with depression.[34]

Trazodone is a triazolopyridine antidepressant that weakly inhibits serotonin reuptake and inhibits alpha (1A and 2C) adrenergic and histamine receptors. The inhibition of histamine and serotonin are thought to be responsible for the sedating effects.[36] In clinical trials, trazodone improved wakening events after sleep onset as well as perceived sleep quality, but did not improve sleep latency or sleep duration.[37] Trazodone is generally well-tolerated, with headache, dry mouth, morning sedation, blurred vision, and gastrointestinal discomfort as the most common reported adverse effects in doses used for insomnia. Higher doses used for depression have been associated with cardiac effects (QTc prolongation, orthostatic hypotension, and syncope), priapism, and serotonin syndrome (particularly when combined with other serotonergic agents).[38,39] Trazodone is not FDA approved for insomnia and there is little evidence about its use in critically ill patients. Although generally well-tolerated, the potential anticholinergic and cardiac effects should be considered in patients with preexisting cardiovascular issues or those receiving other medications with QT prolongation potential.

Mirtazapine is a tetracyclic antidepressant that antagonizes presynaptic alpha-2 adrenergic receptors and postsynaptic serotonin 5-HT2 and 5-HT3 receptors, resulting in an increased release of norepinephrine and serotonin. Mirtazapine also antagonizes the histamine H1 receptor with high affinity, causing significant sedative effects.[40] The sedative properties are particularly relevant at lower doses ($\leq$15 mg) because it is more selective for serotonin and histamine at these doses.[41] It is available in an oral disintegrating tablet, which may be useful in patients with swallowing difficulties. The most common adverse effects are dry mouth and daytime sedation. Additionally, mirtazapine is known to increase appetite and cause weight gain, often being selected for this effect when treating depression.[40] Although rare, cardiac effects such as QT prolongation and arrythmias have occurred been reported in overdose.[41,42]

The tertiary TCAs (doxepin, amitriptyline, trimipramine, clomipramine, and imipramine) are the most sedating owing to their high affinity for the H1 and muscarinic M1 receptors.[43] They decrease the time to sleep onset and improve wakefulness. Secondary TCAs (nortriptyline and desipramine) do not affect these measures.[34] Like other antidepressants, anticholinergic effects (blurred vision, constipation, dry mouth, urinary retention) may be significant. TCAs are also associated with significant cardiac effects, including orthostatic hypotension, QT prolongation, and various arrythmias and cardiac conduction disturbances, especially in the setting of overdose.[43] Seizures have also been reported with cyclic antidepressants and seem to be related directly to dose.[44]

Doxepin has the highest affinity for the H1 receptor among all cyclic antidepressants. It is the only TCA that is FDA approved for insomnia. Doxepin doses used for sleep (3–10 mg) are much lower than doses used for depression (25–300 mg/d) because it is more selective for histamine receptor antagonism at lower doses.[45,46] The half-life of doxepin is approximately 15 hours, which may explain the sleep maintenance benefits observed in clinical trials even late into the final quarter of the night.[24] Its clearance is largely dependent on the CYP2D6 enzyme; monitoring for potential drug interactions is important.

## ANTIPSYCHOTICS

Antipsychotics, most notably quetiapine and olanzapine, are commonly used in the ICU setting in the evening. Data suggest that haloperidol in single doses may increase sleep efficiency and stage 2 sleep, but has little effect on REM sleep.[47] Atypical antipsychotics may increase total sleep time and deep sleep.[47] Although expert consensus remains unclear regarding the usefulness of antipsychotics on sleep promotion, they are viewed as being beneficial in managing delirium that may be impeding sleep (ie, agitation or "sundowning"). If used, it is important to monitor for QTc prolongation with all antipsychotic agents, especially in patients on concomitant medications that may also prolong the QT interval. Haloperidol and olanzapine can be administered parenterally if required. The PADIS guidelines do not make a recommendation regarding the use of antipsychotics for sleep. It is also important to note that the PADIS guidelines also do not recommend the routine use of antipsychotics for the treatment of delirium, but do note their usefulness in the treatment of acute agitation where the patient poses a risk to themselves or others.[8] Antipsychotic therapy, if used, should be discontinued immediately after resolution of agitation and other sleep promotion therapies should be considered.

## ANTIHISTAMINES

Antihistamines are the most common ingredient in over-the-counter sleep aids. Sedation is caused by postsynaptic H1 receptor antagonism.[45] Diphenhydramine and doxylamine are the 2 FDA-approved over-the-counter antihistamines for sleep promotion. First-generation antihistamines (diphenhydramine, chlorpheniramine, hydroxyzine, and doxylamine) cross the blood–brain barrier, unlike the second- and third-generation antihistamines (loratadine, cetirizine, and fexofenadine) which are significantly less sedating. Although there is substantial experience with these agents, postsynaptic muscarinic antagonism may cause significant anticholinergic effects such as dry mouth, blurred vision, urinary retention, and decreased gastrointestinal motility, which can contribute to confusion, delirium, and falls in older adults.[48] Daytime drowsiness is another common deterrent. Additionally, tolerance may develop and limit the prolonged usefulness of these agents.[45]

## SUMMARY

The identification and treatment of sleep disruption in critically ill patients is a persistent and elusive subject. There are many different options for treatment including nonpharmacologic and pharmacologic, with most practitioners using a combination approach. It is important to be cognizant of the multitude of factors that may contribute to impaired sleep in critically ill patients and to address as many of these causes as possible while still carrying out necessary ICU activities and care. Although nonpharmacologic measures are recommended in all patients, the most appropriate pharmacologic agent should be selected based on patient-specific characteristics (ie, patient-reported effectiveness, drug interactions, and disease state interactions). An understanding of the mechanism and safety profiles of pharmacologic agents are imperative in creating safe and multipronged approaches to improve sleep for critically ill patients.

## CLINICS CARE POINTS

- Sleep in the ICU is frequently disrupted by critical illness, interventions, and routine care.

- Nonpharmacologic and pharmacologic therapy should be used together to optimize sleep and address causative factors.
- The choice of pharmacologic therapies should be based on patient- and disease-specific factors.

## DISCLOSURE

The authors have nothing to disclose.

## REFERENCES

1. Delaney LJ, Van Haren F, Lopez V. Sleeping on a problem: the impact of sleep disturbance on intensive care patients - a clinical review. Ann Intensive Care 2015;26:3.
2. Pulak L, Jensen L. Sleep in the intensive care unit: a review. J Intensive Care Med 2016;31:14–23.
3. Honarmand K, McKinley S, Bosma KJ. A systematic review of risk factors for sleep disruption in critically ill adults. Crit Care Med 2020;48:1066–74.
4. Friese RS. Sleep and recovery from critical illness and injury; a review of theory, current practice, and future directions. Crit Care Med 2008;36(3):697–705.
5. Pisani MA, Friese RS, Gehlbach BK, et al. Sleep in the intensive care unit. Am J Respir Crit Care Med 2015;191:731–8.
6. Romagnoli S, Villa G, Fontanarosa L, et al. Sleep duration and architecture in non-intubated intensive care unit patients: an observational study. Sleep Med 2020; 70:79–87.
7. Morales DV, Ballard RD. Sleep and the critically ill patient. In: Lee-Chiong TL, Sateia MJ, Carskadon MA, editors. Sleep Medicine. 2005;32(2):339–47.
8. Devlin JW, Skrobik Y, Gelinas C, et al. Clinical Practice Guidelines for the prevention and management of pain agitation/sedation, delirium, immobility and sleep disruption in adult patients in the ICU. Crit Care Med 2018 Sep;46(9):e825–73.
9. Le Guen M, Nicolas-Robin A, Lebard C, et al. Earplugs and eye masks vs routine care prevent sleep impairment in post-anesthesia care unit: a randomized study. Br J Anaesth 2014;112(1):89–95.
10. Van Rompaey B, Elseviers MM, Van Drom W, et al. The effect of earplugs during the night on the onset of delirium and sleep perception: a randomized control trial in intensive care patients. Crit Care 2012;16(3):R73.
11. Edvardsen JB, Hetmann F. Promoting sleep in the intensive care unit. SAGE Open Nurs 2020;6. 2377960820930209.
12. Shilo L, Dagan Y, Smorjik Y, et al. Effect of melatonin therapy to improve nocturnal sleep in critically ill patients: encouraging results from a small randomized controlled trial. Crit Care 2008;12(2):R52.
13. Product information: circadian oral prolonged-release tablets, melatonin oral prolonged-release tablets. Reading (United Kingdom): RAD Neurim Pharmaceuticals EEC Limited (per EMA); 2017.
14. Product Information: ROZEREM(TM) TABLETS, ramelteon tablets. Lincolnshire (IL): Takeda Pharmaceuticals America, Inc.; 2005.
15. Fontaine G, Der Nigoghossian C, Hamilton LA. Melatonin, ramelteon, suvorexant, and dexmedetomidine to promote sleep and prevent delirium in critically ill patients. Crit Care Nurs Q 2020;43(2):232–50.

16. Bourne RS, Mills GH, Minelli C. Melatonin therapy to improve nocturnal sleep in critically ill patients: encouraging results from a small randomised controlled trial. Crit Care 2008;12:R52.
17. Ibrahim MG, Bellomo R, Hart GK, et al. A double-blind placebo controlled randomised pilot study of nocturnal melatonin in tracheostomized patients. Crit Care Resusc 2006;8:187–91.
18. Tiruvoipati R, Mulder J, Haji K. Improving sleep in intensive care unit: an overview of diagnostic and therapeutic options. J Patient Exp 2019;7(5):697–702.
19. Product Information, package insert: Diprivan intravenous injection, propofol intravenous injection. Fresenius Kabi (per FDA); 2014.
20. Lewis SR, Schofield-Robinson OJ, Alderson P, et al. Propofol for the promotion of sleep in adults in the intensive care unit. Cochrane Database Syst Rev 2018;(1):CD012454.
21. Kondili E, Alexopoulou C, Xirouchaki N, et al. Effects of propofol on sleep quality in mechanically ventilated critically ill patients: a physiological study. Intensive Care Med 2012;38(10):1640–6.
22. Product Information: Precedex(TM) intravenous injection, dexmedetomidine HCl intravenous injection. Lake Forest (IL): Hospira, Inc. (per FDA); 2016.
23. Alexopoulou C, Kondili E, Diamantaki E, et al. Effects of dexmedetomidine on sleep quality in critically ill patients: a pilot study. Anesthesiology 2014;121(4):801–7.
24. Wu XH, Cui F, Zhang C, et al. Low-dose dexmedetomidine improves sleep quality pattern in elderly patients after noncardiac surgery in the intensive care unit: a pilot randomized controlled trial. Anesthesiology 2016;125(5):979–91.
25. Oto J, Yamamoto K, Koike S, et al. Sleep quality of mechanically ventilated patients sedated with dexmedetomidine. Intensive Care Med 2012;38(12):1982–9.
26. Schwartz TL, Goradia V. Managing insomnia: an overview of insomnia and pharmacologic treatment strategies in use and on the horizon. Drugs Context 2013;2013:212257.
27. Lie JD, Tu KM, Shen DD, et al. Pharmacological treatment of insomnia. PT 2015;40(11):759–68, 771.
28. Campanelli CM. American Geriatrics Society updated Beers criteria for potentially inappropriate medication use in older adults. J Am Geriatr Soc 2012;60(4):616–31.
29. Fraser GL, Devlin JW, Worby CP, et al. Benzodiazepine versus nonbenzodiazepine-based sedation for mechanically ventilated, critically ill adults: a systematic review and meta-analysis of randomized trials. Crit Care Med 2013;41(9 Suppl 1):S30–8.
30. Product Information: Sonata®, zaleplon. Philadelphia: Wyeth Laboratories; 1999.
31. Product Information: AMBIEN(R) oral tablets, zolpidem tartrate oral tablets. Bridgewater (NJ): Sanofi-Aventis US LLC (per FDA); 2018.
32. Product Information: LUNESTA™ oral tablet, eszopiclone. Marlborough (MA): Sepracor Inc; 2004.
33. Huedo-Medina TB, Kirsch I, Middlemass J, et al. Effectiveness of non-benzodiazepine hypnotics in treatment of adult insomnia: meta-analysis of data submitted to the Food and Drug Administration. BMJ 2012;345:e8343.
34. Buysse DJ, Tyagi S. Clinical pharmacology of other drugs used as hypnotics. In: Kryger MH, Roth T, Dement WC, editors. Principles and practices of sleep medicine. 6th edition. St Louis, (MO): Elsevier Saunders; 2016. p. 432.
35. Everitt H, Baldwin DS, Stuart B, et al. Antidepressants for insomnia in adults. Cochrane Database Syst Rev 2018;(5):CD010753.

36. Product Information: OLEPTRO(TM) extended-release oral tablets, trazodone hydrochloride extended-release oral tablets. Dublin (Ireland): Labopharm Europe Limited; 2010.
37. Walsh JK, Erman M, Erwin CW, et al. Subjective hypnotic efficacy of trazodone and zolpidem in DSM-III-R primary insomnia. Hum Psychopharmacol 1998; 13:191.
38. Yi XY, Ni SF, Ghadami MR, et al. Trazodone for the treatment of insomnia: a meta-analysis of randomized placebo-controlled trials. Sleep Med 2018;45:25–32.
39. Rao R. Serotonin syndrome associated with trazodone. Int J Geriatr Psychiatry 1997;12(1):129–30.
40. Product Information: REMERON(R) oral tablets, mirtazapine oral tablets. Whitehouse Station (NJ): Merck Sharp & Dohme Corp (per FDA); 2020.
41. Croom KF, Perry CM, Plosker GL. Mirtazapine: a review of its use in major depression and other psychiatric disorders. CNS Drugs 2009;23(5):427–52.
42. Anttila SA, Leinonen EV. A review of the pharmacological and clinical profile of mirtazapine. CNS Drug Rev 2001;7(3):249–64.
43. Anderson IM, Ferrier IN, Baldwin RC, et al. Evidence-based guidelines for treating depressive disorders with antidepressants: a revision of the 2000 British Association for Psychopharmacology guidelines. J Psychopharmacol 2008;22(4): 343–96.
44. Nelson JC. Tricyclic and tetracyclic drugs. In: Schatzberg AF, Nemeroff CB, editors. The American Psychiatric Association Publishing textbook of psychopharmacology. 5th edition. Arlington (VA): American Psychiatric Association Publishing; 2017. p. 305.
45. Krystal AD, Richelson E, Roth T. Review of the histamine system and the clinical effects of H1 antagonists: basis for a new model for understanding the effects of insomnia medications. Sleep Med Rev 2013;17(4):263–72.
46. Rojas-Fernandez CH, Chen Y. Use of ultra-low-dose (<=6 mg) doxepin for treatment of insomnia in older people. Can Pharm J (Ott) 2014;147(5):281–9.
47. Gimenez S, Clos S, Romero S, et al. Effects of olanzapine, risperidone and haloperidol on sleep after a single oral morning dose in healthy volunteers. Psychopharmacology (Berl) 2007;190(4):507–16.
48. American Geriatrics Society Beers Criteria R Update Expert Panel. American Geriatrics Society 2019 updated AGS beers criteria R for potentially inappropriate medication use in older adults. J Am Geriatr Soc 2019;67(4):674–94.

# The Nexus Between Sleep Disturbance and Delirium Among Intensive Care Patients

Lori J. Delaney, RN, MIHM, MN, PG Dip ICU[a,b,c],*,
Edward Litton, MD, PhD[d,e,1], Frank Van Haren, MD, PhD[b,f]

## KEYWORDS

• Delirium • Intensive care • Light • Noise • Sleep • Sleep disturbance

## KEY POINTS

- Sleep disturbance and delirium have a variety of negative sequelae having an impact on patient outcomes, inclusive of physiologic and somatic effects. It is unclear, however, if sleep disturbance leads to delirium, or if delirium is the precipitating cause of sleep disturbance among intensive care patients.
- The bidirectional relationship between sleep disturbance and delirium may be attributed to their neurobiological effects, which have an impact on the function of the prefrontal cortex.
- Neurohormonal changes exhibited in sleep disturbance and delirium are identified to affect the dopaminergic systems, leading to alterations in acetylcholine levels, which are important for attention, motor activity, and memory.
- Nonpharmacologic interventions that have endeavored to address sleep disturbance may have a concurrent positive effect on reducing incidences and duration of delirium, because they seek to normalize the sleep-wake patterns through reduced exposure to light and noise disturbance.
- Effective clinical management for both sleep disturbance and delirium may require a combination of interventions to reduce the adverse effects of the clinical environment, whereby the regulation and normalization of sleep-wake patterns may exert important clinical effects in reducing incidences of delirium.

[a] School of Nursing, Queensland University of Technology, Victoria Park Road, Kelvin Grove, Queensland 4059, Australia; [b] Medical School, Australian National University, Acton 2601, Australian Capital Territory, Australia; [c] Institute of Health and Biomedical Innovation, Musk Avenue, Kelvin Grove, Queensland 4059, Australia; [d] Intensive Care Unit, Fiona Stanley Hospital, Perth, Western Australia 6150, Australia; [e] Intensive Care Unit, St John of God Hospital Subiaco, Perth, Western Australia 6608, Australia; [f] Intensive Care Unit, Department of Intensive Care, Canberra Hospital, Yamba Drive, Garran, Australian Capital Territory 2605, Australia
[1] Present address: Department of Intensive Care Medicine, Royal Perth Hospital, Perth, Western Australia 6000, Australia.
* Corresponding author.
*E-mail address:* lori.delaney@qut.edu.au

Crit Care Nurs Clin N Am 33 (2021) 155–171
https://doi.org/10.1016/j.cnc.2021.01.001
0899-5885/21/© 2021 Elsevier Inc. All rights reserved.

## INTRODUCTION

Intensive care units (ICUs) provide advanced clinical care to support critically ill patients. Inherently, the ICU environment subjects patients to an inordinate amount of clinical monitoring and a panoply of stimuli that frequently are reported to be disruptive and stressful to patients. The implications of this manifests as disturbance to sleep, with research demonstrating high degrees of sleep fragmentation and atypical sleep architecture (structural organization of sleep). Intensive care–based sleep research indicates that 50% of patients report sleep disturbance, with 30% experiencing persistent sleep disturbance post–ICU discharge.[1]

Sleep disturbance has been linked to a variety of negative sequelae, including decreased respiratory function, altered cardiovascular responses, impaired immunologic function, increased pain and anxiety, and decreased overall patient outcomes.[1–3] Factors linked to sleep disturbance within ICUs are diverse and primarily center around the environmental burden and soundscape that patients are subjected to. Research attempting to address these factors has reported varied outcomes, with few studies reporting a sustained benefit in the regulation of the environmental burden and, in turn, enhanced sleep quality.[4–6]

Emerging from current intensive care research is the impact delirium has on patient recovery, with research aimed at improving sleep quality exhibiting positive effects in reducing the incidence and duration of delirium. These findings suggest that there may exist a bidirectional relationship between sleep disturbance and delirium,[7,8] premised on the alterations identified in cognitive function and the positive effects reported in the regulation of sleep-wake patterns.[7,8]

Delirium is reported to complicate 25% of hospital admissions, with incidences as high as 50% among surgical patients, and is disproportionately prevalent among patients cared for in ICUs (20% to 87%).[9–12] The sequelae of delirium is prognostically significant and includes protracted hospital length of stay (up to 10 days) and long-term disability related to activities of daily living.[13,14] Although delirium is considered an acute condition, cognitive function may not be recovered fully, with research indicating that up to 52% of patients do not return to baseline cognitive function,[15] and as many as 25% have impairments comparable to mild Alzheimer disease.[13,16] Delirium in ICU also has been associated with long-term symptoms of posttraumatic stress disorder.[17,18] Reported risk survival analysis suggests delirium does not increase short-term mortality[19,20]; however, the presence of delirium may have an adverse impact on long-term outcomes in which mortality rates appear to be increased. A cohort study conducted by Pisani and colleagues[21] investigating the long-term effects of delirium reported a reduction in 1-year survival by approximately 10% per day of delirium, after adjustment for covariates, such as age, severity of illness, medication, and comorbidities. Both sleep disturbance and delirium are contemporary and challenging issues encountered within the ICU setting that adversely affect patient outcomes. This clinical review analyzes the shared characteristics between sleep disturbance and delirium, addressing pathophysiology, clinical characteristics, and interventions, whereby strategies to address sleep disturbance may exert a beneficial effect on reducing delirium.

## SLEEP DISTURBANCE IN INTENSIVE CARE

Sleep is a complex and dynamic state that is essential for survival. Sleep disturbance among ICU patients is prevalent and considered a contributing factor to the development of delirium. Polysomnography studies involving ICU patients consistently identify the presence of abnormal sleep architecture and atypical electroencephalographic activity, characterized by a predominance of wakefulness and light stages of sleep (stages N1 and N2) (**Fig. 1**). In contrast, the critical restorative stages of sleep; slow wave sleep (SWS) and rapid eye movement (REM) sleep, which are important for mental well-being and physiologic health, are reported to be severely restricted and at times absent.[8,22–25] The acquired total sleep time reported among ICU patients is variable, ranging between 2.1 hours and 8.8 hours, and is highly fragmented, traversing day and night, with circadian dysrhythmia an elevated risk.[22–25] In older adults (aged >60 years), sleep duration normally is reduced and becomes more fragmented, with increased duration of stage N1 (transition stage from wake to sleep) and stage N2 (light sleep) and an accompanying reduction in SWS and REM sleep. These physiologic changes to sleep architecture increase with age and are important to consider in the context of an ICU admission and, in turn, heighten the susceptibility for sleep fragmentation and may exacerbate the propensity to develop delirium. The impact of the interaction between sleep disturbance and delirium remains unclear, although they appear to share similar physiologic features. Fitzgerald and colleagues[26] suggest that significant sleep disturbance is attributed to active delirium, with studies identifying sleep disturbance being a characteristic present in 73% to 99% of patients with delirium.[27,28] The ability to monitor sleep in the ICU remains clinically challenging due to limited feasible options and the gold standard of sleep monitoring, polysomnography, being costly, highly technical, and impractical for widespread implementation. Staff-based observations, although easily implemented,

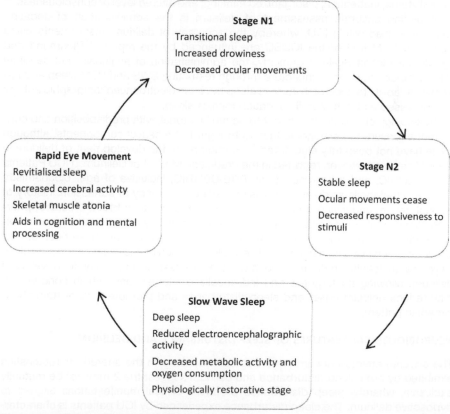

**Stage N1**
Transitional sleep
Increased drowsiness
Decreased ocular movements

**Rapid Eye Movement**
Revitalised sleep
Increased cerebral activity
Skeletal muscle atonia
Aids in cognition and mental processing

**Stage N2**
Stable sleep
Ocular movements cease
Decreased responsiveness to stimuli

**Slow Wave Sleep**
Deep sleep
Reduced electroencephalographic activity
Decreased metabolic activity and oxygen consumption
Physiologically restorative stage

**Fig. 1.** Physiologic characteristics of the sleep cycle.

nonintrusive, and cost-effective, are deemed subjective and inaccurate to inform clinical decision making, with research indicating that staff overestimate the duration of sleep and are unable to effectively report the extent of sleep fragmentation.[2,29]

## DELIRIUM IN INTENSIVE CARE

A diagnosis of delirium presents as a clinical challenge due to its variable clinical presentation and manifestation of symptoms. According to the *Diagnostic and Statistical Manual of Mental Disorders* (Fifth Edition),[30] delirium is characterized by an acute onset of impaired awareness and attention, which can be accompanied by disturbance in cognition and exhibits a fluctuating course (hours to days). Three phenotypes of delirium—hypoactive, hyperactive, and mixed delirium—have been reported, with hyperactive states easily identified due to their symptoms.[31] In contrast, hypoactive and mixed delirium are more challenging to identify and, without defined assessments, can go unrecognized or misdiagnosed. The Confusion Assessment Method (CAM)–ICU or the Intensive Care Delirium Screening Checklist (ICDSC) commonly are used within ICUs to assess for the presence of delirium. The psychometric properties of the ICDSC report a high level of sensitivity (99%), with a lower specificity of 64%, which may result in the misclassification of conditions leading to a misdiagnosis of delirium.[32] In contrast, the CAM-ICU has been validated within a larger ICU population, is less subjective than the ISDSC, and allows for rapid assessment (approximately 2 minutes to complete) evaluating 4 domains: acute onset of changes in mental status, inattention, disorganized thinking, and altered level of consciousness.[33] Confounding accurate assessment of delirium is the administration of sedation commonly used within ICU, whereby the accuracy of delirium assessments using either the CAM-ICU or the ICDSC are influenced by the reported Richmond and Agitation-Sedation Scale.[34] Similarly, the administration of analgesia and sedation has an impact on sleep architecture through restricting SWS and REM sleep and impedes the ability to accurately assess sleep because electroencephalographic activity is suppressed and behaviorally sedation mimics sleep.

The etiology of delirium is thought to be multifactorial, with predisposition and concurrent exposure to deliriogenic factors thought to be causal components, although these have not been fully elucidated.[35] Predictors for the development of delirium in the ICU setting, however, reported in the Prediction Model For Delirium in ICU Patients (PRE-DELIRIC) and the revised Early PRE-DELIRIC, inclusive of age, biochemistry (urea and metabolic acidosis), admission category, urgency of admission, history of alcohol abuse, underlying cognitive impairment, mean arteria blood pressure, pharmacologic agents (corticosteroids, morphine, and sedative administration), and respiratory failure at the time of or within 24 hours of ICU admission, have been shown accurate predictive assessments.[36] The implementation of this assessment may allow clinicians to identify patients who have the greatest susceptibility to developing delirium, allowing for targeted and individualized interventions, which concurrently may reduce delirium onset and sleep disturbance and promote a more normalized circadian pattern.

## NEUROBIOLOGICAL FEATURES OF SLEEP DISTURBANCE AND DELIRIUM

The adverse effects outwardly manifested secondary to the shared characteristics exhibited by both sleep disturbance and delirium suggest the 2 may not be mutually exclusive, whereby sleep disturbance produces clinical manifestations aligned to hypoactive delirium. The sleep disturbance experienced by ICU patients is characterized by restricted SWS and REM sleep, inducing a sleep debt with a concomitant increase in sleep pressure. This produces clinical manifestations of daytime somnolence, impaired cognition (memory and attention), altered mood, and circadian dyssynchrony, which reflect the salient features of delirium.[37] The neurocognitive dysfunctions demonstrated in sleep disturbance and delirium share similar recovery timelines, in which compromised psychomotor vigilance associated with sleep disturbance can be reversed with 3 nights to 5 nights of unrestricted sleep.[38] This recovery timeframe to restore neurobehavioral function is reflective of that reported in delirium.[38]

Neurobiological research has identified shared neurohormonal effects of delirium and sleep disturbance on the brain. Delirium exerts its effects on the cerebral cortex and brainstem affecting the prefrontal cortex, parietal lobes, and basal ganglia, which are important for attention and working memory.[37] Sleep deprivation produces altered electroencephalographic activity indicative of suboptimal prefrontal cortical functioning.[39,40] The neurobiological effects exerted as a result of sleep disturbance impede cerebral glucose metabolic rate in the parietal cortex and thalamus, which has an adverse impact on the modulation of alertness and cognitive performance.[39,41]

The neurohormonal changes exhibited in both sleep disturbance and delirium are suggested as secondary to alterations in the dopaminergic systems, primarily related to a reduction in acetylcholine levels.[42] The neurochemical factors contributing to delirium are putatively an impairment in cerebral oxidative metabolism attributed to a decrease in cholinergic neurotransmitters and a concurrent increase in dopaminergic activity.[43] Acetylcholine plays a significant role in the interaction with dopamine, which is deemed important for attention, motor activity, and memory.[43,44] Research suggests that acetylcholine levels are reduced in REM sleep deprivation, whereas K-complexes are reduced in SWS and are considered important sleep characteristics, which aid in the consolidation of memory.[45] The dopaminergic dysregulation present in delirium is inadvertently regulated by the administration of antipsychotics, which inhibits dopamine release and balances the dopamine and cholinergic responses.[26] These medications appear to have limited beneficial effect on sleep architecture, however, through increasing stage N2 sleep and minimal effect on increasing restorative sleep phases (SWS and REM sleep).[46]

The suppression of the neurohormone melatonin is attributed to both the pathogenesis of delirium and sleep disturbance. The risk factors associated with the onset of delirium, such as underlying dementia, age, and medications, are linked to altered pleiotropic melatonergic functions (**Fig. 2**).[26] Melatonin plays a critical role in the regulation of circadian rhythms, sleep, mood, immune response, and aging.[47,48] The role of melatonin and its pharmacologic potential is of particular interest within intensive care due to its role in sleep and the reported suppression of melatonin levels in critically ill patients.[49,50] Shigeta and colleagues[51] identified abnormal melatonin secretion was present among patients who developed postoperative delirium, suggesting that postoperative alterations resulting in the disturbance of the sleep-wake patterns may precipitate the onset of delirium. The administration of supplemental melatonin is being explored and prefaced as an intervention to address primarily sleep and circadian disturbance; concomitantly, it also may play an important role in decreasing the incidence of delirium via a negative feedback system, which reduces serotonin and tryptophan catabolism.[52]

## THE EFFECTS OF ANALGESIA AND SEDATION ON SLEEP AND DELIRIUM

The administration of sedation and analgesia is an integral component to patient care within the ICU, although a paradigm shift has occurred with regard to the quantities

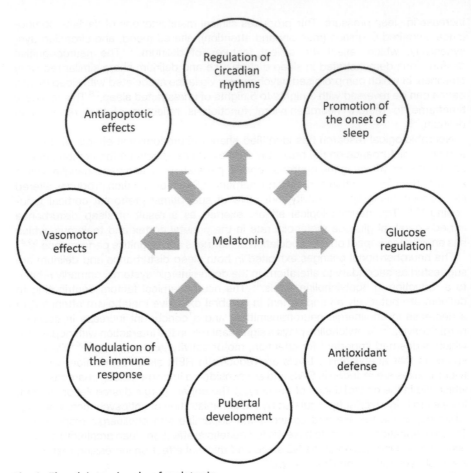

**Fig. 2.** The pleiotropic role of melatonin.

and types of pharmacologic agents used in order to reduce adverse effects linked to their administration: increased risk of infection, pressure injuries, enteral nutrition intolerance, mechanical ventilation, and ICU length of stay.[53] Sedation has established effects on the sleep architecture and development of delirium through the suppression of SWS and REM sleep due to the inhibition of γ-aminobutyric acid (GABA) and Mu-opioid receptors (**Fig. 3**).[54] GABA and Mu-opioid receptor agonists readily cross the blood-brain barrier, exerting an anticholinergic effect, and are associated with the development of delirium.[55,56] Research suggests that the administration of GABA agonists, such as propofol and benzodiazepines, is increased during the night (23:00 hours–07:00 hours) among patients receiving mechanical ventilation[57] and further impedes the excretion of melatonin.[58–60] Zaal and colleagues[61] attributed the administration of benzodiazepines to an increased risk and causal factor for delirium among intensive care patients. The increased use of sedative medications overnight indicates a potential misalignment between sedation assessment and perceived patient needs, knowledge deficits, and erroneous beliefs that the use of sedation promotes patient sleep. Rather, increased administration of benzodiazepines restricts REM sleep and may compromise cerebral blood flow.[57,62–64] As a result, there is a call for a more

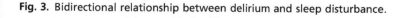

| Delirium | Sleep disturbance |
|---|---|
| Effects neurological function | Effects neurological function |
| Adversely impacts on sleep continuity | Linked to the onset of delirium |
| Presents with diffuse cognitive deficits | Produces diffuse cognitive deficits |
| Altered GABA activity effecting sleep-wake cycle | Altered melatonin levels resulting in altered sleep-wake cycles |
| Benzodiazepine adminstration increases risk delirium | Administration of benzodiazepines to faciliate sleep restricts SWS and REM sleep |
| Limiting environmental burden reduces incidences of delirium | Reducing environmental burden improves subjective sleep quality |

**Fig. 3.** Bidirectional relationship between delirium and sleep disturbance.

judicious approach to the selection and administration of sedatives prescribed to intensive care patients, with a greater emphasis on targeted and monitored sedation scores.

In an effort to reduce daily administration amounts of sedatives, identification of alternative medication choices, such as $\alpha_2$-adrenergic agonists (eg, dexmedetomidine), increasingly are considered. Dexmedetomidine, which exerts several functions, inclusive of sedation, analgesia, and sympatholytic effects, has emerged as a potential option that minimises disruption to normal sleep architecture.[57,65] Comparably, dexmedetomidine has demonstrated favorable effects in the treatment of delirium.

Findings of the Dexmedetomidine to Lessen ICU Agitation study suggests that dexmedetomidine, compared with a placebo or standard care, reduced mechanical ventilation time and time to extubation and resulted in a reduction in the duration of delirium.[66] Dexmedetomidine may exert a beneficial effect on sleep architecture, with research involving healthy participants indicating an increase in SWS, and did not adversely affect psychomotor vigilance.[67] Intensive care–based studies investigating dexmedetomidine's ability to improve sleep report an increase in the percentage of stage N2 sleep, improved sleep efficiency and subjective sleep quality, and a reduction in the percentage of stage N1 sleep.[68] The emergence of such findings proffers dexmedetomidine as a viable sedative option that may aid in reducing the need and administration of benzodiazepines. Restricting the administration of benzodiazepines would have a concurrent beneficial impact on sleep architecture, because they impede SWS and REM sleep, produce an increase in stage N2 sleep, increase daytime somnolence, and have an adverse impact on psychomotor vigilance.[67,69] Paradoxically, benzodiazepine administration may contribute to insomnia, hallucinations, and increased agitation.[70] The effect of dexmedetomidine on sleep quality appears to yield a favorable effect on normalizing sleep-wake patterns and increases sleep efficiency but does not rectify the abnormal sleep architecture reported among ICU patients,[65,71,72] highlighting the intricacies related to pharmacologic agents' impact on both sleep and delirium and how addressing one of these issues may inadvertently influence the other.

## NONPHARMACOLOGIC INTERVENTIONS
### Reducing Environmental Burden

#### Light
The intensive care setting imposes an environmental constancy throughout the 24-hour period, which is not conducive to quietude and obscures the distinction between day and night. Research endeavoring to address the issues of environmental burden to improve sleep concurrently has reported reductions in the incidence and duration of delirium within the intensive care setting. As a result, these nonpharmacologic interventions have formed a basis for specific and bundled interventions in an attempt to improve sleep within the ICU (**Fig. 4**).

Light exposure has a significant impact on circadian patterns secondary to the human eyes' photosensitive retinal ganglion cells, which communicate with the suprachiasmatic nucleus and act as the circadian pacemaker.[73] The ICU environment obfuscates this zeitgeber (external cue to entrain biological rhythms) secondary to the prolonged exposure to artificial lighting. The luminance levels within the ICU are reported to range between 5 lux and 1400 lux, whereby low luminance levels (<500 lux) for 20 minutes can result in a suppression of melatonin levels.[74,75]

Research attempting to address the issues attributed to restricted exposure to natural light levels suggest that use of bright light therapy (>1500 lux) may have a beneficial effect in reducing the need for pharmacologic intervention,[76–78] and incidences of delirium among postoperative patients.[79,80] Potharajaroen and colleagues[78] identified that the combination of bright light exposure in conjunction with oxygen therapy may provide a preventative effect for delirium, secondary to maintaining sleep-wake cycles and stabilizing bicarbonate levels. Understanding the impact of clinical design appears to be an important consideration when attempting to address both sleep disturbance and delirium, whereby the absence of visible daylight is reported to increase the risk of developing delirium (odds ratio 2.39),[81] compared with single-room access and enhanced daylight exposure, which are reported to reduce the

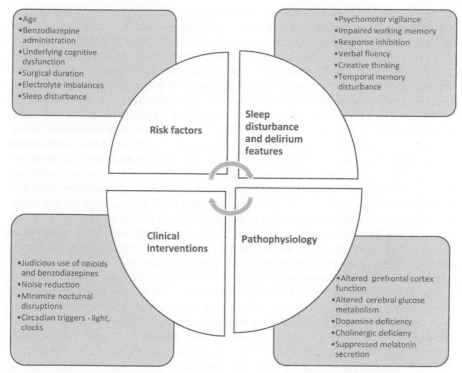

- Age
- Benzodiazepine administration
- Underlying cognitive dysfunction
- Surgical duration
- Electrolyte imbalances
- Sleep disturbance

- Psychomotor vigilance
- Impaired working memory
- Response inhibition
- Verbal fluency
- Creative thinking
- Temporal memory disturbance

**Risk factors**

**Sleep disturbance and delirium features**

**Clinical interventions**

**Pathophysiology**

- Judicious use of opioids and benzodiazepines
- Noise reduction
- Minimize nocturnal disruptions
- Circadian triggers - light, clocks

- Altered prefrontal cortex function
- Altered cerebral glucose metabolism
- Dopamine deficiency
- Cholinergic deficieny
- Suppressed melatonin secretion

**Fig. 4.** The comparative clinical characteristics and findings shared between delirium and sleep disturbance.

duration of delirium and concurrently improved sleep quality.[80] As a result, consideration to chronobiological clinical design features may contribute to improve sleep-wake cycles, while providing a more normalized day-night environment, leading to a reduction in incidences and duration of delirium and sleep disturbance.

Chronobiological research undertaken in the ICU to improve sleep quality largely has focused on addressing the impact of the clinical environment, primarily light and noise exposure; however, reported findings largely have been subjective and have not translated into long-term improvements within the ICU. The adjunct findings in many of these studies is the impact that amendments to the environment have on the incidence and duration of delirium, which reiterates the contention of a bidirectional relationship between sleep and delirium.

### Noise

The soundscape of the ICU environment is diverse and highly variable, with noise intensity significantly higher than recommended by the World Health Organization.[82] The complexity of the clinical environment and the accompanying intensive monitoring and their associated alarms are the primary contributors to the adverse soundscape. Noise has been identified as a factor that frequently is attributed to sleep disturbance in the ICU setting, with research indicating that noise reduction improved patients perceived sleep quality. Biophysiologic research of sleep and patient responsiveness to nocturnal acoustical variations, however, indicates that sleep may not be disrupted primarily by noise events, with previous studies employing polysomnography indicating that noise levels were only able to be attributed to 11% to 25% of sleep arousals.[22,24]

This suggests that there may be additional contributing factors, such as clinical interactions, neurohormonal changes, and altered physiologic responses to critical illness, that lead to sleep disturbance and, in turn, may precipitate the onset of delirium.

Noise reduction studies have focused on behavior and environmental modifications and sound masking. Behavioral modifications, such as adjusting alarm volumes for a nocturnal environment, making staff more cognizant of conversations and volume of speech occurring in proximity of patients, closing patient doors, and implementing noise-absorbing furnishings, have reported subjective reductions in perceived noise and improved patients' reported sleep quality.[83] The ability to sustain the implemented practices remains untested, however, with physiologic measures of sound and sleep being limited. The use of sound-masking strategies, such as earplugs, has been reported to have beneficial effects on sleep quality, along with reducing confusion and onset of delirium.[84] Van Rompaey and colleagues[84] demonstrated a risk reduction in the development of delirium by 53% (hazard ratio 0.47; 95% CI, 0.27–0.82), combined with a concurrent improvement in subjective sleep quality ($P$ = .042). Findings such as these have been reiterated by Le Guen and colleagues,[85] who reported an improvement in sleep quality assessed via the Spiegel scale, with a reduction in disorientation with the concurrent implementation of earplugs and eye masks in postoperative patients ($P$ = .01). Furthermore, quality improvement initiatives, such as those by Kamdar and colleagues,[5] also have highlighted the potential positive effect of mitigating noise exposure via the use of earplugs and background music to improve sleep, which resulted in a reduction in subjective noise ratings ($P$ = .001) and incidence of delirium ($P$ = .02).[5] In a meta-analysis conducted by Litton and colleagues,[86] the implementation of earplugs significantly reduced risk of delirium (risk reduction 0.59; 95% CI, 0.44–0.78), and beneficially the intervention was minimally invasive and cost-effective to implement. Despite these findings, the widespread use and implementation of earplugs and ear masks remain largely unadopted, due to a lack of recognized benefit in their implementation among patients requiring sedation and mechanical ventilation. Concerns regarding the additional sensory deprivation that eye masks and earplugs provide and their impact on patient autonomy, particularly when cognitive disturbances are present, may be confounding factors for both staff and patients relating to their wider adoption as a component of care.[87]

Understanding the impact of noise abatement interventions can be challenging due to the variable approaches used to assess and quantify noise and its impact, because many studies do not employ environmental noise monitoring or polysomnography to monitor sleep; rather, they evaluate noise levels and sleep quality via subjective assessments. Noise abatement strategies, such as earplugs, appear to have a variable effect on sleep quality and quantity; rather, they may provide beneficial clinical effects in reducing anxiety and administration of sedatives,[88,89] both of which can negatively affect sleep via reducing restorative sleep phases (SWS and REM sleep), whereby impaired sleep quality may precipitate the onset of delirium. These suggest that potentially clinicians need to be more attuned to the environmental burden and soundscape of the ICU in relation to its impact on patients. The ability to sustain the positive effect of noise reduction strategies frequently has been challenged, however, because behavioral and cultural practice changes in the ICU require a prolonged and focused approach in order for these to be adopted as normalized practice. In addition, the design of the ICU has an effect on behavior in terms of noise reverberations, and how staff interact within the space, such as locations of nursing stations, utility rooms, workflow, and shared patient care spaces, are factors that may limit the effect and success of noise abatement interventions.

*Bundle interventions*

The Society of Critical Care Medicine Clinical Practice Guidelines for the Prevention and Management of Pain, Agitation/Sedation, Delirium, Immobility, and Sleep Disruption in Adult Patients in the ICU[90] advocate for a multicomponent approach to sleep, because studies indicate a multifaceted approach aids in reducing delirium incidences and concurrently promotes sleep.[90,91] Approaches, such as quiet time interventions, offer patients a potential reprieve from the constant nature of the ICU environment, quiet time interventions are defined as spans of time in which clinical interactions are purposely reduced along with noise and light levels to promote periods of rest. Although the time of day to schedule quiet times is debated, there is a growing body of research that suggests that they has a positive effect on sleep quality,[92,93] with Olson and colleagues[92] reporting an increase in observed sleep behavior 1.6 times greater than in those receiving standard care. Van de Pol and colleagues[94] found sleep to be unaffected by the implementation of a quiet time intervention, although the need for sleep-inducing medication was significantly reduced ($P<.001$). The intervention was found to facilitate a decrease in noise levels ($P = .02$), with a reduced need for pharmacologic intervention proposed as a contributing factor in the concurrent reduction in delirium ($P = .02$). Intuitively, approaches aimed an ameliorating the clinical environment appear to offer some benefit to patients and establish a more patient-centered approach in which sleep may be more likely to be acquired. This, in combination with less physiologic stress related to the soundscape and intensity of the clinical care, may have a synergistic effect in reducing the need for pharmacologic intervention and its impact on sleep architecture and, in turn, reduces the susceptibility to delirium. The contribution of each of the components that comprise a bundled intervention, however, has not been explored sufficiently, resulting in variances in interventions coined quiet time intervention. The intention of quiet time interventions also is susceptible to being derailed and becoming a time where clinical staff can address care needs and interventions that they may not have had the opportunity to undertake at alternate times, inadvertently making the designated period more aligned to staff and workflow needs rather than a patient-centered intervention. The physiologic benefit of quiet time interventions may be debated in that few studies implement the gold standard for sleep monitoring, polysomnography, to ascertain the biophysiologic effect such interventions have on sleep architecture, opting for subjective assessment or proxy measures of sleep quality.

In a randomized controlled study, Boyko and colleagues,[93] sought to identify if improvements in the ICU clinical environment, yielded through a quiet time protocol, inclusive of restricted visitation, limiting diagnostic procedures and treatments conducted between 22:00 hours to 06:00 hours, and reduced alarm volumes and luminance exposure, in combination with the implementation of eye masks and earplugs, resulted in increased sleep quality assessed via polysomnography. The study demonstrated a reduction in environmental noise, albeit not a statistically significant reduction ($P = .3$), and no evidence that quiet time improved sleep among mechanically ventilated patients ($P = .7$).[93] The findings of the study are limited due to its low recruitment numbers (n = 17) and the limited number of polysomnography (53%; n = 9) studies that exhibited physiologic characteristics of normal sleep, highlighting the complexity of monitoring and interpreting sleep within the ICU patient population, who frequently exhibit pathologic encephalographic activity. As a result, the impact and contribution of intrinsic factors, such as inflammatory mediators and neurobiological changes in response to critical illness, combined with pain and effects of commonly infused pharmacologic agents to provide sedation and analgesia cannot be discounted for sleep disturbance and as causal factors for delirium. This in part may account for the positive effects that are yielded by studies administering supplemental melatonin due to its pleiotropic effects.

As a result, the effect of quiet time interventions remains inconclusive and appears to have some beneficial impact in reducing environmental burden but not definitively in promoting sleep. Rather, it may provide a rest period that provides patients with a reduction in stimulus and the need for medication to limit patient responsiveness to their clinical environment. Interventions that address several considerations that have an adverse impact on sleep appear to be more successful in improving subjective sleep quality and in turn may have beneficial impact on delirium, rather than single isolated interventions. This approach integrates various interventions, such as curbing noise exposure through behavior modification and use of earplugs and eye masks to limit intrusive light during the nocturnal phase, earlier mobilization and activity during the day, clustered care, and pharmacologic review. Implementing a multidisciplinary bundle, Patel and colleagues[94] demonstrated an increase in sleep efficiency ($P = .031$) and a concomitant reduction in noise levels ($P = .002$), reduction luminance ($P = .003$), and reduction in delirium ($P<.001$). A bundled approach primarily targets factors attributed to sleep disturbance, although these may not translate to improved biophysiologic characterization of sleep. There do appear to be some favorable benefits in terms of reduced environmental burden and potentially incidence and duration of delirium. As a result, the relationship between sleep and delirium requires further research and clinical evaluation to ascertain the impact of interventions.

## SUMMARY

Sleep disturbance remains a complex issue in the ICU and may have an important link to the onset and duration of delirium and vice versa. The concurrent neurophysiologic effects demonstrate considerable similarities, exerting effects on the cortex and brainstem. Alterations in the secretion of neurotransmitters and hormonal regulation that are critical in maintaining normal circadian patterns appear present in both delirium and sleep disturbance, potentially exacerbated by the administration of pharmacologic agents commonly prescribed in the ICU setting. The ability to distinguish between the primary effects of sleep disturbance and delirium remains unclear; however, as research evolves, there appears to be a consolidation of the ideas that sleep disturbance may be a causative factor for delirium. Understanding these effects is critical, because delirium has been demonstrated to increase morbidity, mortality, and length of ICU stay. As a result, monitoring sleep and sleep promotion need to be integrated as standard components of clinical care for intensive care patients.

## CLINICS CARE POINTS

- Judicious administration of GABA and mu-opioid receptor agonists is needed because these have an adverse impact on sleep architecture, sleep-wake cycles, and psychomotor vigilance. Limiting the administration of benzodiazepines in preference for dexmedetomidine may have a beneficial effect on normalizing sleep patterns, improving sleep quality, and reducing incidences of delirium.

- A multifaceted clinical approach aimed at normalizing wake-sleep cycles is beneficial in regulating circadian patterns and reducing adverse effects related to sleep disturbance and delirium.

- Being cognizant of the environmental burden imposed by an intensive care admission is necessary to recognize and respond to the stimuli that may impede sleep and contribute to the development of delirium.

- Nonpharmacologic interventions, such as bundled interventions and quiet time approaches, may be preferrable in the management of delirium, because the use of antipsychotics fails to support a normal sleep architecture and SWS and REM sleep.

## DISCLOSURE

The authors have nothing to disclose.

## REFERENCES

1. Beltrami FG, Nguyen XL, Pichereau C, et al. Sleep in the intensive care unit. J Bras Pneumol 2015;41:539–46.
2. Delaney LJ, Van Haren F, Lopez V. Sleeping on a problem: the impact of sleep disturbance on intensive care patients - a clinical review. Ann Intensive Care 2015;5:3.
3. Salas RE, Gamaldo CE. Adverse effects of sleep deprivation in the ICU. Crit Care Clin 2008;24:461–76.
4. Jones C, Dawson D. Eye masks and earplugs improve patient's perception of sleep. Nurs Crit Care 2012;17:247–54.
5. Kamdar BB, King LM, Collop NA, et al. The effect of a quality improvement intervention on perceived sleep quality and cognition in a medical ICU. Crit Care Med 2013;41:800–9.
6. Li SY, Want TJ, Wu SF, et al. Efficacy of controlling night-time noise and activities to improve patients' sleep quality in a surgical intensive care unit. J Clin Nurs 2011;20:396–407.
7. Flannery AH, Oyler DR, Weinhouse GL. The impact of interventions to improve sleep on delirium in the ICU: a systematic review and research framework. Crit Care Med 2016;44(12):2231–40.
8. Pisani MA, Friese RS, Gehlbach BK, et al. Sleep in the intensive care unit. Am J Respir Crit Care Med 2015;191(7):731–8.
9. Pisani MA, Murphy TE, Van Ness PH, et al. Characteristics associated with delirium in older patients in a medical intensive care unit. Arch Intern Med 2007;167(15):1629–34.
10. Girard TD, Pandharipande PP, Ely EW. Delirium in the intensive care unit. Crit Care 2008;12:S3.
11. Dasgupta M, Dumbrell AC. Perioperative risk assessment for delirium after noncardiac surgery: a systemic review. J Am Geriatr Soc 2006;54:1578–89.
12. Norbert Z, Coburn M. Acute confusional states in hospital. Dtsch Arztebl Int 2019;116:7.
13. Shi Q, Presutti R, Selchen D, et al. Delirium in acute stroke: a systematic review and meta-analysis. Stroke 2012;43:645–9.
14. Sato K, Kubota K, Oda H, et al. The impact of delirium on outcomes in acute, non-intubated cardiac patients. Eur Heart J Acute Cardiovasc Care 2017;6:553–9.
15. Cole MG, Bailey R, Bonnycastle M, et al. Partial and no recovery from delirium in older hospitalized adults. J Am Geriatr Soc 2015;63:2340–8.
16. Pandharipande PP, Girard TD, Jackson JC, et al. Long-term cognitive impairment after critical illness. N Engl J Med 2013;369:1306–16.
17. Brück E, Schandl A, Bottai M, et al. (2018). The impact of sepsis, delirium, and psychological distress on self-rated cognitive function in ICU survivors—a prospective cohort study. J Intensive Care 2018;6(1):1–8.

18. Bulic D, Bennett M, Georgousopoulou EN, et al. Cognitive and psychosocial out-
    comes of mechanically ventilated intensive care patients with and without
    delirium. Ann Intensive Care 2020;10:104.
19. Duprey MS, van den Boogaard M, van der Hoeven JG, et al. Association between
    incident delirium and 28- and 90-day mortality in critically ill adults: a secondary
    analysis. Crit Care 2020;24(1):161.
20. Klein Klouwenberg PM, Zaal IJ, Spitoni C, et al. The attributable mortality of
    delirium in critically ill patients: prospective cohort study. BMJ 2014;349:g6652.
21. Pisani MA, Kong SY, Kasl SV, et al. Days of delirium are associated with 1-year
    mortality in an older intensive care unit population. Am J Respir Crit Care Med
    2009;180:1092–7.
22. Gabor J, Cooper A, Crombach S, et al. Contribution of the intensive care unit
    environment to sleep disruption in mechanically ventilated patients and healthy
    subjects. Am J Respir Crit Care Med 2003;167:708–15.
23. Elliott R, McKinley S, Cistulli P, et al. Characterisation of sleep in intensive care
    using 24-hour polysomnography: an observational study. Crit Care 2013;
    17(2):R46.
24. Freedman NS, Gazendam J, Levan L, et al. (2001). Abnormal sleep/wake cycles
    and the effect of environmental noise on sleep disruption in the intensive care
    unit. Am J Respir Crit Care Med 2001;163(2):451–7.
25. Friese RS, Diaz-Arrastia R, McBride D, et al. (2007). Quantity and quality of sleep
    in the surgical intensive care unit: are our patients sleeping? J Trauma 2007;
    63(6):1210–4.
26. Fitzgerald JM, Adamis D, Trzepacz PT, et al. Delirium: a disturbance of circadian
    integrity? Med Hypotheses 2013;81(4):568–76.
27. Meagher DJ, Moran M, Raju B, et al. Phenomenology of delirium: assessment of
    100 adult cases using standardised measures. Br J Psychiatry 2007;190(2):
    135–41.
28. Mattoo SK, Grover S, Chakravarty K, et al. Symptom profile and etiology of
    delirium in a referral population in northern India: factor analysis of the DRS–
    R98. J Neuropsychiatry Clin Neurosci 2012;24(1):95–101.
29. Delaney LJ, Van Haren F, Currie M, et al. Sleep monitoring techniques within
    intensive care. Int J Nurs Clin Pract 2015;2:114–9.
30. American Psychiatric Association. Diagnostic and statistical manual of mental
    disorders (DSM-5®). Arlington, VA: American Psychiatric Pub; 2013.
31. Krewulak K, Stelfox HT, Leigh JP, et al. Incidence and prevalence of delirium sub-
    types in an adult ICU: a systematic review and meta-analysis*. Crit Care Med
    2018;46(12):2029–35.
32. Bergeron N, Dubois MJ, Dumont M, et al. Intensive care delirium screening
    checklist: evaluation of a new screening tool. Intensive Care Med 2001;27:
    859–64.
33. Figueroa-Ramos MI, Arroyo-Novoa CM, Lee KA, et al. Sleep and delirium in ICU
    patients: a review of mechanisms and manifestations. Intensive Care Med 2009;
    35:781–95.
34. van den Boogaard M, Wassenaar A, van Haren FM, et al. Influence of sedation on
    delirium recognition in critically ill patients: a multinational cohort study. Aust Crit
    Care 2020;33(5):420–5.
35. Jenewein J, Büchi S. The neurobiology and pathophysiology of delirium. Schweiz
    Arch Neurol Psychiatr 2007;158:360–7.
36. Wassenaar A, Schoonhoven L, Devlin JW, et al. External validation of two models
    to predict delirium in critically ill adults using either the confusion assessment

method-ICU or the intensive care delirium screening checklist for delirium assessment. Crit Care Med 2019;47(10):e827–35.

37. Durmer JS, Dinges DF. Neurocognitive consequences of sleep deprivation. Semin Neurol 2005;25:117–25.

38. Lamond N, Jay SM, Dorrian J, et al. (2007). The dynamics of neurobehavioural recovery following sleep loss. J Sleep Res 2007;16(1):33–41.

39. Lowe CJ, Safati A, Hall PA. The neurocognitive consequences of sleep restriction: a meta-analytic review. Neurosci Biobehav Rev 2017;80:586–604.

40. Smith ME, McEvoy LK, Gevins A. The impact of moderate sleep loss on neurophysiologic signals during working memory task performance. Sleep 2002;25:784–9.

41. Thomas ML, Sing HC, Belenky G, et al. Neural basis of alertness and cognitive performance impairments during sleepiness II. Effects of 48 and 72 h of sleep deprivation on waking human regional brain activity. Thalamus Relat Syst 2003;3:199–229.

42. Ebert D, Albert R, Hammon G, et al. Eye-blink rates and depression: is the antidepressant effect of sleep deprivation mediated by the dopamine system? Neuropsychopharmacology 1996;15(4):332–9.

43. Trzepacz PT. Update on the neuropathogenesis of delirium. Dement Geriatr Cogn Disord 1999;10:330–4.

44. Trzepacz PT. In there a final common neural pathway in delirium? Focus on acetylcholine and dopamine. Semin Clin Neuropsychiatry 2000;5:132–48.

45. Benedito MAC, Camarini R. Rapid eye movement sleep deprivation induces an increase in acetylcholinesterase activity in discrete rat brain regions. Braz J med Biol Res 2011;34(1):103–9.

46. Gimenez S, Clos S, Romero S, et al. Effects of olanzapine, risperidone and haloperidol on sleep after a single oral morning dose in healthy volunteers. Psychopharmacology 2007;190:507–16.

47. Brzezinski A. Melatonin in humans. N Engl J Med 1997;16:186–95.

48. Reiter RJ. Pineal melatonin: cell biology of its synthesis and of its physiological interactions. Endocr Rev 1991;12:151–80.

49. Golombek DA, Rosenstein RE. Physiology of circadian entrainment. Physiol Rev 2010;90(3):1063–102.

50. Bourne RS, Mills GH. Melatonin: possible implications for the postoperative and critically ill patient. Intensive Care Med 2006;32(3):371–9.

51. Shigeta H, Yasui A, Nimura Y, et al. Postoperative delirium and melatonin levels in elderly patients. Am J Surg 2001;182:449–54.

52. Balan S, Leibovitz A, Zila SO, et al. The relation between the clinical subtypes of delirium and the urinary level of 6-SMT. J Neuropsychiatry Clin Neurosci 2003;15:363–6.

53. Bawazeer M, Amer M, Maghrabi K, et al. Adjunct low-dose ketamine infusion vs standard of care in mechanically ventilated critically ill patients at a Tertiary Saudi Hospital (ATTAINMENT Trial): study protocol for a randomized, prospective, pilot, feasibility study. Trials 2020;21:288.

54. Bourne RS, Mills GH. Sleep disruption in critically ill patients-pharmacologic considerations. Anaesthesia 2004;59:374–84.

55. Pandharipande P, Ely EW. Sedative and analgesic medications: risk factors for delirum and sleep disturbances in the critically ill. Crit Care Clin 2006;22:313–27.

56. Roche V. Southwestern internal medicine conference. Etiology and management of delirium. Am J Med Sci 2003;325:20–30.

57. Seymour CW, Pandharipande PP, Koestner T, et al. Diurnal sedative changes during intensive care: impact on liberation from mechanical ventilation and delirium. Crit Care Med 2012;40:2788–96.
58. McIntyre IM, Norman TR, Burrows GD, et al. Human melatonin response to light at different times of the night. Psychoneuroendocrinology 1989;14(3):187–93.
59. Govitrapong P, Pariyanonth M, Ebadi M. The presence and actions of opioid receptors in bovine pineal gland. J Pineal Res 1992;13:124–32.
60. Frisk U, Olsson J, Nylen P, et al. Low melatonin excretion during mechanical ventilation in the intensive care unit. Clin Sci 2004;107(1):47–53.
61. Zaal IJ, Devlin JW, Hazelbag M, et al. (2015). Benzodiazepine-associated delirium in critically ill adults. Intensive Care Med 2015;41(12):2130–7.
62. Weinert CR, Calvin AD. Epidemiology of sedation and sedation adequacy for mechanically ventilated patients in a medical and surgical intensive care unit. Crit Care Med 2007;35(2):393–401.
63. Kajimura N, Nishikawa M, Uchiyama M, et al. Deactivation by benzodiazepine of the basal forebrain and amygdala in normal humans during sleep: a placebo-controlled [15O]H2O PET study. Am J Psychiatry 2004;161(4):748–51.
64. Weinhouse GL, Watson PL. Sedation and sleep disturbances in the ICU. Crit Care Clin 2009;25(3):539–49.
65. Lu W, Fu Q, Luo X, et al. (2017). Effects of dexmedetomidine on sleep quality of patients after surgery without mechanical ventilation in ICU. Medicine 2017; 96(23):e7081.
66. Reade MC, Eastwood GM, Bellomo R, et al. Effect of dexmedetomidine added to standard care on ventilator-free time in patients with agitated delirium: a randomized clinical trial. JAMA 2016;315(14):1460–8.
67. Akeju O, Hobbs LE, Gao L, et al. (2018). Dexmedetomidine promotes biomimetic non-rapid eye movement stage 3 sleep in humans: a pilot study. Clin Neurophysiol 2018;129(1):69–78.
68. Wu XH, Cui F, Zhang C, et al. Low-dose dexmedetomidine improves sleep quality pattern in elderly patients after noncardiac surgery in the intensive care unit: a pilot randomized controlled trial. Anesthesiology 2016;125(5):979–91.
69. Daou M, Telias I, Younes M, et al. Abnormal sleep, circadian rhythm disruption, and delirium in the ICU: are they related? Front Neurol 2020;11:1089.
70. Mistraletti G, Carloni E, Cigada M, et al. Sleep and delirium in the intensive care unit. Minerva Anestesiol 2008;74(6):329–34.
71. Oto J, Yamamoto K, Koike S, et al. (2012). Sleep quality of mechanically ventilated patients sedated with dexmedetomidine. Intensive Care Med 2012; 38(12):1982–9.
72. Alexopoulou C, Kondili E, Diamantaki E, et al. Effects of dexmedetomidine on sleep quality in critically Ill patients: a pilot study. Anesthesiology 2014;121(4): 801–7.
73. Vethe D, Scott J, Engstrøm M, et al. The evening light environment in hospitals can be designed to produce less disruptive effects on the circadian system and improve sleep. Sleep 2020;zsaa194. https://doi.org/10.1093/sleep/zsaa194.
74. Boivin DB, Duffy JF, Kronauer RE, et al. Dose response relationship for resetting of human circadian clock by light. Nature 1996;379:540–2.
75. Drouot X, Cabello B, Ortho M, et al. Sleep in the intensive care unit. Sleep Med Rev 2008;12:391–403.
76. Yang J, Choi W, Ko YH, et al. Bright light therapy as an adjunctive treatment with risperidone in patients with delirium: a randomized, open, parallel group study. Gen Hosp Psychiatry 2012;34(5):546–51.

77. Chong MS, Tan KT, Tay L, et al. (2013). Bright light therapy as part of a multicomponent management program improves sleep and functional outcomes in delirious older hospitalized adults. Clin Interv Aging 2013;8:565.
78. Potharajaroen S, Tangwongchai S, Tayjasanant T, et al. (2018). Bright light and oxygen therapies decrease delirium risk in critically ill surgical patients by targeting sleep and acid-base disturbances. Psychiatry Res 2018;261:21–7.
79. Taguchi T, Yano M, Kido Y. Influence of bright light therapy on postoperative patients: a pilot study. Intensive Crit Care Nurs 2007;23(5):289–97.
80. Ono H, Taguchi T, Kido Y, et al. The usefulness of bright light therapy for patients after oesophagectomy. Intensive Crit Care Nurs 2011;27(3):158–66.
81. Van Rompaey B, Elseviers MM, Schuurmans MJ, et al. Risk factors for delirium in intensive care patients: a prospective cohort study. Crit Care 2009;13(3):R77.
82. Delaney LJ, Currie MJ, Huang HCC, et al. The nocturnal acoustical intensity of the intensive care environment: an observational study. J Intensive Care 2017; 5(1):41.
83. Kumar S, Ng RQ, Lee HP. Experimental investigations of acoustic curtains for hospital environment noise mitigations. Computer Science, Physics, arXiv: Applied Physics 2020. https://arxiv.org/ftp/arxiv/papers/2008/2008.06690.pdf.
84. Van Rompaey B, Elseviers MM, Van Drom W, et al. The effect of earplugs during the night on the onset of delirium and sleep perception: a randomized controlled trial in intensive care patients. Crit Care 2012;16(3):1–11.
85. Le Guen M, Nicolas-Robin A, Lebard C, et al. Earplugs and eye masks vs routine care prevent sleep impairment in post-anaesthesia care unit: a randomized study. Br J Anaesth 2014;112:89 95.
86. Litton E, Carnegie V, Elliott R, et al. The efficacy of earplugs as a sleep hygiene strategy for reducing delirium in the ICU: a systematic review and meta-analysis. Crit Care Med 2016;44(5):992–9.
87. Simons KS, van den Boogaard M, de Jager CP. Reducing sensory input in critically ill patients: are eye masks a blind spot? Crit Care 2012;16:439.
88. Aydın Sayılan A, Kulakaç N, Sayılan S. The effects of noise levels on pain, anxiety, and sleep in patients. Nurs Crit Care 2020. https://doi.org/10.1111/nicc.12525.
89. Devlin JW, Weinhouse GL. Earplugs, sleep improvement, and delirium: a noisy relationship. Crit Care Med 2016;44(5):1022–3.
90. Devlin JW, Skrobik Y, Gélinas C, et al. (2018). Clinical practice guidelines for the prevention and management of pain, agitation/sedation, delirium, immobility, and sleep disruption in adult patients in the ICU. Crit Care Med 2018;46(9):e825–73.
91. Devlin JW, Skrobik Y, Gelinas C, et al. Executive summary: clinical practice guidelines for the prevention and management of pain, agitation/sedation, delirium, immobility, and sleep disruption in adult patients in the ICU. Crit Care Med 2018;46:1532–48.
92. Olson DM, Borel CO, Laskowitz DT, et al. Quiet time: a nursing intervention to promote sleep in neurocritical care units. Am J Crit Care 2001;10(2):74–8.
93. Boyko Y, Jennum P, Nikolic M, et al. Sleep in intensive care unit: the role of environment. J Crit Care 2017;37:99–105. 005.
94. van de Pol I, van Iterson M, Maaskant J. Effect of nocturnal sound reduction on the incidence of delirium in intensive care unit patients: an interrupted time series analysis. Int Crit Care Nur 2017;41:18–25.

# The Impact of Obstructive Sleep Apnea on the Sleep of Critically Ill Patients

Michaelynn Paul, RN, DNP, CCRN-K

## KEYWORDS

- Sleep • Sleep apnea • Obstructive sleep apnea • Critical care • Intensive care

## KEY POINTS

- Obstructive sleep apnea is often undiagnosed.
- Obstructive sleep apnea can have deleterious impacts on the critically ill patient.
- Education is necessary for critical care staff.
- Early identification and intervention can improve patient outcomes.

## INTRODUCTION

The economic impact of sleep deprivation is staggering. In 2017, it was reported that, combined, the United States, UK, Germany, Japan, and Canada lost upwards of $680 billion in each of the 5 years studied.[1] Workplace productivity in the United States alone was decreased by an equivalent of 1.23 million working days owing to sleep deprivation. This lack of sleep leads to an increase in mortality risk of 13% in individuals who averaged fewer than 6 hours of sleep per night. Clearly, sleep deprivation is costly. It has been estimated that 80% of critically ill patients experience the consequences of sleep deprivation.[2] The recognition of the impact of lack of sleep on critically ill patients is drawing attention to the prevalence of this issue and the need for a solution.

The causes of sleep loss are multifactorial; however, one of the most prevalent causes is obstructive sleep apnea (OSA).[3] OSA is not only associated with daily functional impairment, but also leads to a decreased quality of life. Combined with multiple comorbidities, such as cardiovascular disease and obesity, sleep deprivation related to OSA is increasing in prevalence worldwide.

## THE IMPACT OF SLEEP DEPRIVATION AND OBSTRUCTIVE SLEEP APNEA COMORBIDITIES

The impact of sleep deprivation is significant on a healthy person, but can be compounded in a patient who is critically ill and has diagnosed OSA.[2,3] Further

Walla Walla University, School of Nursing, 10345 Southeast Market Street, Portland, OR 97216, USA
E-mail address: Michaelynn.Paul@wallawalla.edu

Crit Care Nurs Clin N Am 33 (2021) 173–192
https://doi.org/10.1016/j.cnc.2021.01.009
0899-5885/21/© 2021 Elsevier Inc. All rights reserved.

compounding care may be undiagnosed OSA. The combination of lack of sleep and OSA can disrupt many body systems and impact the healing for the critically ill hospitalized patient. A thorough understanding of the causes of lack of sleep in combination with the comorbidities, and risk factors of OSA will lead to the development of specific interventions to mitigate complications and enhance patient outcomes.

## COMORBIDITIES, RISK FACTORS, AND ASSOCIATED BODY SYSTEMS
### Inflammation and Endocrine Function

Sleep deprivation is known to significantly impact the immune system causing the body to be more susceptible to infections when proinflammatory cytokines are increased in the bloodstream.[4] This increase in cytokines along with systemic inflammation lowers the body's defense mechanisms.[5] In a multicenter trial of 73 male patients, of whom 26 had moderate to severe OSA, several factors were identified that predicted OSA. In these patients, glycated hemoglobin (P<.001), C-reactive protein (P<.001), and erythropoietin (P<.05) were significantly higher than their counterparts without OSA. The combination of glycated hemoglobin and C-reactive protein predicted the probability of moderative to severe OSA 92% of the time.[6]

Sleep deprivation leads to increased cortisol levels, increased C-reactive protein, plasma tumor necrosis factor-alpha, and IL-10.[7] Increased glucocorticoid levels, corticotropin-releasing hormone, and adrenocorticotropic hormone lead to hyperactivation of the hypothalamic–pituitary–adrenal axis, leading to poor endocrine function.[8] There is an association between sleep deprivation and type 2 diabetes.[9] This association may be due in part to intermittent hypoxemia from sleep apnea and sleep deprivation, which leads to pancreatic cellular dysfunction and insulin resistance.[10] One study demonstrated a reciprocal association between diabetes and OSA. In pooled analysis of more than 145,000 patients from 3 cohorts, it was noted that OSA was associated with a 37% higher risk of diabetes and a 43% higher risk of OSA in individuals with diabetes who were also on insulin therapy.[11]

### Respiratory Function

Sleep deprivation leads to difficulty weaning patients from mechanical ventilation owing to depressed responses to carbon dioxide and hypoxia.[12] Decreased inspiratory endurance has been correlated with a decrease in sleep in healthy males, which could result in respiratory failure, particularly in a critically ill patient.[13] Sleep deprivation is also seen in patients with OSA who experience fragmented sleep owing to intermittent hypoxia. In a recent study, patients with OSA and coronavirus disease 2019 (COVID-19) were more likely to be hospitalized (15.3% vs 3.4%; P<.0001) than those who did not have OSA, and were more likely to develop respiratory failure (19.4% vs 4.5%; P<.0001).[14]

### Neurologic Function

Neurocognitive function is significantly impaired by lack of sleep, causing a decrease in the ability to sustain attention, which leads to slower physiologic recovery of cerebral restoration.[15] Sleep deprivation increases the risk of having a stroke.[16] Multiple studies have associated OSA with the prevalence of stroke and noted that, as the severity of OSA increases, so does the incidence of stroke.[17] In 1 study of 794 patients with suspected OSA who were analyzed for stroke, the cumulative incidence of stroke was significantly higher in the severe untreated OSA group (log-rank test, 11.87; P = .01). In a systematic review, with pooled results of 37 studies and 3242 patients, researchers evaluated the prevalence of OSA in patients with cerebrovascular disease.[18] The results indicated a prevalence rate of 70.4% of those with an apnea–hypopnea index (AHI) of greater than 5 and 61.9% of patients with an AHI of greater than 10. In 14 studies including 1298 patients, 30.1% had an AHI of greater than 30.

## Cardiovascular System

Within the cardiovascular system, sleep deprivation leads to endothelial dysfunction, which causes the release of cytokine and growth factors, increased coagulability, increased vasoconstriction, and decreased vasodilator mediators, which lead to cardiovascular complications.[19] Sleep deprivation has been associated with hypertension, heart rate variability, and higher diastolic blood pressure. Those who are sleep deprived have a greater risk of cardiogenic shock, cardiac arrest, and ST segment elevation myocardial infarctions.[20] In a study, that was conducted as a part of the Sleep Heart Health Study, a cohort of 3265 patients were followed for 9.5 years to analyze whether OSA occurring during REM sleep was associated with a composite cardiac end point.[21] The patients with diagnosed cardiovascular disease had higher rates of moderate (31.9% vs 17.5%; $P<.001$) and severe (14.4% vs 8.6%; $P = .013$) OSA during REM sleep. In total, 749 participants had 418 coronary artery disease events (myocardial infarction or coronary revascularization procedure), 233 had heart failure events, and 98 experienced a stroke. A significant number of these events (53.5% vs 18%; $P<.001$) occurred in patients with preexisting cardiovascular disease.

## Obesity

Individuals who are overweight or obese report twice as many sleep problems and, overall, less sleep and poorer quality sleep than their nonobese counterparts.[22] This result is in part due to excessive fat deposits that narrow the airways and decrease respiratory muscular activity. This factor leads to hormonal imbalances, such as decreased melatonin, which alters circadian rhythms and then potentially results in weight gain. Weight gain is also associated with an increase in AHI severity. It was reported in the Wisconsin Sleep Study that a 10% weight gain predicted a 32% increase in the AHI and increased the odds of developing moderate to severe sleep-disordered breathing.[23] Interestingly, Lin and associates[24] reported that the length of the upper airway correlated with body weight. When matched with body mass index (BMI) and the length of the upper airway in the patients with OSA (81.99 ± 5.88 vs 70.19 ± 6.41; $P<.001$), results suggested that body weight played a role in the length of the upper airway.

## Additional Impacts

Finally, sleep deprivation leads to an increased length of stay in the hospital and mortality.[25] Less time spent in REM sleep was associated with an increased risk of all-cause mortality in a cross-sectional study with 2 independent cohorts of more than 4000 patients.[26] A lack of sleep or sleep interruptions have long been associated with the risk of developing delirium.[27] In 1 study, diminished total sleep time and longer latency to sleep onset on the first night in the hospital were associated with more severe delirium on postoperative day 2.[28] The development of delirium increases the length of stay by an average of 1.9 days.[29] Although there are many reasons for critically ill patients to experience sleep deprivation, the focus of this review is to analyze the impact of sleep apnea.

## PREVALENCE OF SLEEP APNEA

The prevalence of OSA is varied throughout the world with some limitations that include ethnic variations and under-represented subpopulations, home testing versus hospital admissions, physician diagnosed versus actual polysomnography (PSG), and reporting overall rates versus rates by severity.[30] Continued analysis is necessary to appreciate the actual prevalence of OSA.

In a systematic review analyzing 24 studies from multiple countries, the prevalence was varied.[30] Overall, prevalence ranged from 9% to 38% for the adult population as measured by an AHI of 5 or higher or a respiratory disturbance index (RDI) of 5 or more events per hour. The prevalence was higher in men (13%–33%) than women (6%–19%) and, in some advanced age groups, it was as high as 84% (90% in men). When analyzing AHI events of 15 or more, the overall prevalence for the adult population was 6% to 17% but again as high as 36% in older populations. A Belgian study was able to complete 1809 home polygraphy studies and showed a prevalence rate of 41% for mild OSA, 11.8% for moderate OSA, and 6.5% for severe OSA.[31] As in the previous systematic review, prevalence was greater in men (two-thirds vs one-third) than women.

The analysis of studies from several vulnerable populations showed similar prevalence rates. A sample of US African Americans enrolled in the Jackson Heart Sleep Study showed that 24% had AHI scores of 15 or higher based on an in-home apnea study using wrist actigraphy.[32] Of those, 95% had not been diagnosed with sleep apnea by a physician. Using data from the 2005 to 2014 National Survey on Drug Use and Health public files, a sample (n = 20,631) showed an average prevalence of sleep apnea at 5.9%; however, it was noted that rates were increasing from 3.7% in 2005 to 8.1% (P for trend = .001 for the adjusted model) at the end of the study in 2014.[33]

In a Norwegian prevalence study of 1887 patients, researchers analyzed the correlation between OSA and multiple acute and chronic conditions, and found that 29.6% had mild OSA, 17.3% had moderate OSA, and 15.2% had severe OSA. Additionally, the prevalence of obesity, diabetes, hypertension, chest pain, and myocardial infarction were significantly increased with greater OSA severity.[34] Lower prevalence rates were reported in a French study of 5146 intensive care unit (ICU) patients, where 289 patients (5.6%) had OSA on admission; however, severity according AHI was not reported. No significant change in length of stay was reported; however, a subgroup (n = 138) who had OSA with a BMI of greater than 40 kg/m$^2$ was associated with a significant increase in length of stay in the ICU (incident rate ratio, 1.56 [95% CI 1.05; 2.32]; P = .03).[35] Similarly, an American study of 150,77 ICU patients showed that 1183 (7.8%) had a diagnosis of OSA on admission. PSG showed an AHI index of more than 5 events per hour in 835 patients (71%) with OSA.[36] Another American study using the Nationwide Inpatient Sample database analyzed 74,032 mechanically ventilated patients with pneumonia and reported a prevalence rate of 10.3% (n = 7620) with OSA.[37] There was no significant difference noted in length of stay (OSA median 11 days vs no OSA median 11 days; P = .68).

## DEFINITION OF SLEEP APNEA

OSA is characterized by reoccurring episodes of obstructed airways, either partial or complete, that occur during sleep and result in apnea or hypopneas.[38,39] Apnea is defined as the complete cessation of airflow and hypopneas are defined as a decrease in airflow of 30% as measured by a nasal pressure transducer.[40] Some researchers propose further research into phenotypes for OSA to further categorize patients by symptoms, response to therapy, health outcomes, and quality of life.[41]

## PATHOPHYSIOLOGY

OSA occurs owing to the upper airway/pharynx partially or completely collapsing repeatedly during sleep.[39,42,43] This collapse occurs behind the base of the tongue and opposite the soft palate causing apnea (a complete collapse) or hypopnea (an incomplete collapse). The patency of the pharynx is maintained during inspiration through the contraction of the dilator muscles. These dilator muscles include the genioglossus muscle, which contracts to keep the posterior portion of the tongue from collapsing during inspiration, the levator and tensor palatini muscles, which elevate and advance the soft palate, and the stylopharyngeus and geniohyoid muscles, which support the lateral pharyngeal walls. There are 3 components central to causing this collapse: narrowing anatomy of the upper airways, neuromuscular control of pharyngeal permeability, and ventilatory control.

Individuals with OSA often have narrowed upper airways owing to deposits of fat in the parapharyngeal fat pads and muscles; however, narrowing can be due to craniofacial structural abnormalities.[39,42,43] These abnormalities might include deviations of soft tissues and/or skeletal structures. Soft tissue abnormalities include a long thick, soft palate and/or a large tongue with posterior or inferior bulging. Skeletal structure abnormalities include an inferiorly positioned hyoid bone, shorter mandibular or maxillary length, or verticalization of the mandible. Together these soft tissues and skeletal structures lead to the narrowing of the posterior pharyngeal and retrovelar spaces which decreases the efficiency of the contracting dilator muscles. Additionally, during sleep, fluid accumulates in the pharyngeal area, which promotes obstruction.[44] This factor is more prevalent in patients who have heart failure, chronic renal failure, and hypertension.

Pharyngeal musculature modulates the caliber of the pharynx.[39,42,43] Neuromuscular compensation causes increased activity of the dilator muscles owing to reduced pharyngeal caliber when the patient wakes up. When the patient falls asleep, there is less activation of these muscles, thus increasing the potential for the dilator muscles to collapse. The risk of this collapse is greater owing to increased resistance of inspiration and expiration from narrowed upper airways. Pharyngeal neuropathy may be caused by increased pharyngeal resistance, which leads to activation of dilator muscles owing to impaired protective reflexes. The cause of pharyngeal neuropathy may be related to denervated lesions from intermittent hypoxia and the vibration of snoring or neuromuscular pathology.

Destabilization of the respiratory control loop is caused by an excessive ventilatory response to frequent nighttime microarousal.[39,42,43] This induces activation of the pharyngeal muscles and cyclical variations in respiratory control. Although these arousals do not normally wake the patient, they do cause daytime sleepiness. This intermittent hypoxemia and hypercapnia during pharyngeal collapse and subsequent increase in intrathoracic pressures leads to stimulation of the sympathetic nervous system, which contributes to hypertension and metabolic complications. Each event leads to chronic adaptation and oxidative stress, inflammation, and remodeling. These conditions lead to the activation of the inflammation cascade, endothelial activation, and increased stiffness of the arterial walls. Nitric oxide production results in increased vasoconstriction, which activates sympathetic hyperactivity and the renin–angiotensin–aldosterone system, which contributes to continued hypertension. Increased catecholamine levels alter lipid, carbohydrate, and hepatic metabolism, which results in decreased sensitivity of insulin owing to the increased flow of free fatty acids to the liver and muscles. Promotion of lipolysis from inflamed fatty tissues leads to an increase in low-density lipoprotein cholesterol, promoting atherogenesis.

## CLINICAL PRESENTATION

The traditional clinical presentation of OSA includes loud or irregular snoring, daytime sleepiness, unrefreshing sleep regardless of sleep duration, increased fatigue related to sedentary status, nocturia, choking and gasping during sleep, dry mouth on awakening, morning headaches, a BMI of greater than 30, a crowded oropharynx, and an increased neck circumference (men >17 inches and women >15 inches).[45] Semelka and associates[46] reported nocturia and snoring, but also stated that snoring increased with the severity of OSA. Additionally, researchers noted the inclusion of the elbow sign, which is described as the bed partner elbowing the snoring individual. Arnold and associates[47] reported similar clinical presentations of OSA; however, used the assessment of neck size of 16 inches or greater in females. Laratta and colleagues[48] noted additional assessments such as morning headaches, poor concentration irritability, erectile dysfunction, bed partners reporting snoring, or witnessed apneas. Miller and Berger[49] added sleep fragmentation and insomnia as presenting symptoms.

Several more current studies validated these findings; however, they also provided additional potential presenting symptoms. In a study of 392 patients where 135 (34%) had moderate to severe OSA (<15), 46% had evening sock marks, 43% reported heavy legs during the day, and 33% had a morning stuffed nose.[50] This was in response to newer information, which suggested that daytime fluid accumulation led to nocturnal fluid shifts, which worsens OSA. A multivariate analysis demonstrated that evening sock marks was an independent correlate of an AHI of greater than 15 along with being male, older, and experiencing self-reported snoring and apneas. Bauters and colleagues[31] noted the following strong associations with mild and moderate to severe OSA: (1) male (odds ratio [OR]), 1.96 (95% confidence interval [CI], 1.41–2.70; $P<.001$); (2) advancing age (OR, 1.95; 95% CI, 1.74–2.16; $P<.001$; per decade increase in age); (3) BMI (OR, 1.87; 95% CI, 1.67–2.07; $P<.001$); and (4) habitual snoring (OR, 1.96; 95% CI, 1.51–2.54; $P<.001$). Of interest in a cross-sectional analysis study of 1009 patients, 29.5% of the study group reported morning headaches (n = 298).[51] Spalka and associates[51] noted, however, that morning headaches were not associated with the severity of OSA.

## ASSESSMENT AND DIAGNOSIS
### Severity Stratification

The AHI, which is the mean number of apneas and hypopneas in 1 hour of sleep, is used to measure disease severity.[52] Using this scale, OSA is defined as mild when the AHI score is more than 5 but less than 15 per hour, moderate when the AHI score is more than 15 but less than 30, and severe when the AHI score is 30 or more and when each stage is also accompanied with daytime sleepiness.[52,53] Some authors have questioned the validity of the AHI; however, it is the current gold standard for measuring the severity of AHI.[53–55]

The AHI is calculated using PSG.[56] PSG uses physiologic assessments from the electroencephalogram, electro-oculogram, electromyogram, electrocardiogram, pulse oximetry, respiratory effort, and airflow during sleep to determine the cause of sleep disorders. Although PSG is the gold standard for measuring AHI, the American Academy of Sleep Medicine recommended in 2018 the inclusion of an arousal-based scoring system, which would quantify respiratory effort-related arousals per hour of sleep.[57] Including the additional criteria has the potential to capture younger, nonobese patients with OSA who would otherwise not have been correctly diagnosed.

The American Academy of Sleep Medicine criteria for hypopnea scoring for adults uses recommended rule 1A or the acceptable rule 1B.[58] The recommended rule 1A scores a respiratory event as a hypopnea if each criteria parameter is met. The 3 criteria include: (1) peak signal excursions drop by 30% or greater of pre-event baseline using nasal pressure, positive airway pressure device flow or an alternative hypopnea sensor, (2) a duration of the 30% or greater decrease if the signal excursion is 10 seconds or longer, and (3) there is a 3% or greater oxygen desaturation from pre-event baseline and/or the event is associated with an arousal. The acceptable rule 1B includes the same first 2 criteria but allows for a 4% or greater oxygen desaturation from the pre-event baseline. Kapur and Donovan[59] suggest adding a respiratory event index to the 3% oxygen desaturation criteria because it would more accurately predict cardiovascular risk.

Unfortunately, many patients admitted to the ICU may never have been tested for OSA and assessment questionnaires may not be able to be appropriately administered to critically ill patients owing to intubation, sedation, or level of consciousness. However, the questionnaires can provide a quick and efficient method of analysis of the potential risk that, in the alert patient, leads to further investigation of the possibility of OSA and thus alters patient outcomes, depending on the results.

### Assessment Questionnaires

The results of screening tests are often reported based on analyzing the sensitivity and specificity as compared with a gold standard.[60] The sensitivity of a screening test is described as the ability of the test to identify a true positive or all the people who have a specific condition. The specificity of a screening test is described as the ability of a test to identify a true negative or all the people who do have the specific condition. The application of sensitivity and specificity testing allows for the accurate interpretation of the results of questionnaires to accurately classify patients.

There are 2 common questionnaires used to screen patients for OSA; however, both have specificity issues. The STOP-BANG questionnaire is a screening tool that consists of 8 items as self-reported by the patient and was originally designed for presurgical patients.[46,61] A high risk of OSA is considered if there is a positive response to 3 or more of the items. The questionnaire has 2 components. First, the STOP component analyzes signs and symptoms of possible OSA, such as snoring, daytime tiredness, observed episodes of apnea during sleep, and high blood pressure. Second, the BANG component analyzes physical features that are associated with the increased risk of developing OSA, and include, BMI of greater than 35 kg/m$^2$, 50 years of age or older, neck size larger than 17 inches in males or 16 inches in females, and male sex.

Previous studies reported sensitivities of more than 85% and specificity ranging between 25% and 85% (noting higher specificity for obese males).[46] Miller and Berger[49] correlated the sensitivity to AHI events. The sensitivity for an AHI of 5 or higher was 83.6%, for an AHI of 15 or higher was 92.3%, and it was 100% for an AHI of 30 or higher. However, they also reported that specificity scores were limited in terms of reliability.

In a more recent study of 100 male commercial drivers, Popevic and associates[62] also compared sensitivity and specificity scores to AHI events. In this study, sensitivity and specificity for greater than 5 AHI events were 86.0% and 53.5%, for greater than 15 events were 100.0% and 40.3%, and for greater than 30 events were 100.0% and 35.2%. The researchers suggested increasing the scoring to 4 positive answers instead of 3 for overall accuracy, indicating that false positives could burden the limited capacities of sleep clinics. Abumuamar and colleagues[63] had similar concerns regarding the lack of good specificity for patients with atrial fibrillation, noting that the sensitivity was good (89%), but that the low specificity (36%) and a high-false positive rate (64%) were problematic. Researchers suggested, in this study, that the questionnaire would miss 11% of patients with OSA and result in administering PSG to 64% of patients who did not have OSA. Therefore, it was recommended that regardless of the results of the questionnaire that level II sleep studies be administered for patients with underlying atrial fibrillation. Nagappa and associates[61] conducted a systematic review and meta-analysis to analyze the validation of the STOP-BANG questionnaire among different populations (renal, sleep clinic, and surgical). Pooled sensitivity and specificity scores for all OSA or an AHI of 5 or greater were 0.90 and 0.51, respectively. For moderate to severe OSA or an AHI of 15 or more, the pooled sensitivity and specificity scores were 0.94 and 0.40, respectively. Finally, for severe OSA or an AHI of 20 or more, the pooled sensitivity and specificity scores were 0.96 and 0.25, respectively.

Although the STOP-BANG questionnaire is the most widely used owing to its ease of administration, there are other screening tools. Prasad and colleagues[64] analyzed 9 screening questionnaires for assessing the likelihood of OSA, which included the Berlin Questionnaire (BQ), the modified Berlin Questionnaire (MBQ), STOP, STOP-BANG, OSA-50, sleep apnea clinical score, Epworth sleepiness scale (ESS), American Society of Anesthesiologists checklist, and the elbow sign questionnaire. The MBQ had the highest sensitivity (92.7%) followed by the STOP-BANG (89%) for prediction of OSA with an AHI of 5 or more. Specificity, however, was 34.8% and 43.5%, respectively. For an AHI of 15 or less, the MBQ had a specificity score of 29.7% and the STOP-BANG had a score of 39.2%.

The ESS, to assess daytime sleepiness, is an 8-item self-reported questionnaire in which patients rate, on a 4-point Likert scale, the likelihood of dozing or falling asleep during 8 different situations.[65] These situations include sitting and reading, watching TV, laying down to rest in the afternoon, sitting and talking to someone, sitting in the car while stopped in traffic, sitting in a public place, as a passenger in a car, and sitting quietly having lunch. A score of 0 to 30 is possible with a score of more than 10 suggesting excessive daytime sleepiness and scores of greater than 16 generally associated with significant sleep disorders.

Senaratna and colleagues[66] determined that, in their study sample of middle-aged individuals with OSA-related symptoms, the ESS used in combination with other OSA screening tools (STOP-BANG and OSA-50) could increase the specificity from between 21 - 59% to 92 - 95%, but at the expense of sensitivity. Additionally, this combination of screening tools missed more than 50% of individuals with clinically relevant OSA. The researchers did create a decision support tool using the STOP-BANG and ESS cutoff scores and their corresponding ability to detect clinically relevant OSA; however, this tool would require further validation.

Guo and colleagues[67] conducted a study to determine if weighting the components of the EES questionnaire would improve accuracy of the predicting AHI events. Two prospective cohorts, derivation (n = 756) and validation (n = 810), were used to support the weighted ESS. The weighted EES provided increased correlation with AHI events through improved sensitivities and specificity scores when compared with non-weighted ESS. Normal daytime sleepiness indicated a sensitivity of 100% with an associated specificity of 85%; mild excessive daytime sleepiness showed 92.3% and 90.2% sensitivity and specificity, respectively; moderate excessive daytime sleepiness 58.5% and 83.6%; and severe excessive daytime sleepiness 59% and 98%. The weighted ESS would likely detect the difference between patients with simple snoring versus patients with OSA and improve avoidance of expensive PSG and decrease the burden on sleep centers.

The BQ is 10 questions within 3 different categories.[68] In the first category, information is gathered regarding snoring severity; in category 2, daytime somnolence; and in category 3, the presence of hypertension and/or a BMI of more than 30 kg/m$^2$.[2] Risk for OSA is defined if 2 or more categories are positive. Ng and colleagues[69] evaluated 316 patients in 2 groups to analyze the predictive accuracy of the BQ in patients with suspected OSA undergoing PSG with those undergoing home diagnoses through the Embletta portable diagnostic system at home. The prevalence of moderate to severe OSA in the sample was 54%. Of those, the BQ identified 99 patients (69.7%) in the home group and 100 (77.5%) in the hospitalized group. This translated to a sensitivity and specificity of 78% and 23% to predict an AHI of 15 or higher, leading researchers to suggest the Berlin test was not reliable in predicting OSA with PSG and the AHI from normal participants without OSA.

Tan and associates[70] conducted a similar study with 242 patients and found that 79 (32.6%) were classified as high risk according to the BQ with a sensitivity and specificity of 58.8% and 77.6% for predicting an AHI 15 or more events and improved its sensitivity to 76.9% for an AHI of 30 or greater; however, there was a corresponding decrease in the specificity to 72.7%. Finally, Wu and colleagues[71] analyzed the potential interference of pulmonary function on the performance of the BQ, MBQ, and STOP-BANG scores when screening for OSA in patients with chronic obstructive pulmonary disease. All 3 tests performed well; however, they were more accurate with a lower forced expiratory volume in 1 second percent predicted or forced vital capacity percent predicted value. The BQ showed a sensitivity and specificity of 53% and 89%, respectively; the MBQ was 65% and 85%, respectively; and the STOP-Bang was 84% and 59%, respectively. Clearly, there are issues with each of the screening tools; however, in terms of efficiency the STOP-BANG questionnaire continues to be the most widely used screening tool.

## POLYSOMNOGRAPHY

PSG remains the gold standard laboratory-based diagnostic test to monitor both sleep and respiratory parameters.[39] PSG is noninvasive and monitors multiple physiologic parameters related to sleep and wakefulness through simultaneous recordings.[39,72] To analyze the assessment of sleep stages electroencephalography, electro-oculography, and surface electromyography are used. Two electroencephalography channels with ear references are used to monitor sleep latency and arousals. Two electro-oculography channels monitor the horizontal and vertical eye movements to document the onset of sleep and rapid eye movement sleep. The electromyography channel records skeletal muscle movement or the lack thereof with electrodes over the chin, mentalis, or submentalis. Airflow can be monitored through the nose or the mouth to measure the presence or absence of airflow using a thermistor channel. Pressure transducers are more sensitive to restrictions of airflow and evaluating hypopneas. Additional parameters that are measured include electrocardiography, pulse oximetry, thoracic and abdominal respiratory effort (through the use of resistance bands), end-tidal carbon dioxide levels, surface electromyography monitoring for leg and arm movements, and video monitoring.[72]

## TREATMENT
### Behavioral

By the time the patient is in the ICU, behavioral options are not going to be immediately effective. However, a stay in the ICU may act as a motivator for future change. Most behavioral changes include regular aerobic exercise, weight loss, avoiding supine sleeping, and abstinence from alcohol.[39] In a recent study, 86 patients were given 10 individual sessions with a dietician and a physiotherapist regarding behavior modifications.[73] The experimental group received a behavioral sleep medicine intervention that focused on enhanced physical activity and good nutrition. Although the number of participants in each group was small, the experimental group (n = 14) moved from severe to moderate OSA to moderate to mild versus the control group (n = 6; P = .02). Multivariate analyses indicated that odds were 4.5 times higher (after adjusting for baseline AHI and amount of body fat) for improvement of OSA category. This finding indicates that exercise should be included in any behavioral modification program.

In analyzing the role of weight management in the treatment of OSA, Hudgel and associates[74] created an evidenced based guideline. A summary of their guidelines, as they relate to diet and exercise, suggests participation in a comprehensive lifestyle program, which includes eating fewer calories, increasing activity, and behavioral counseling. For patients with a BMI of 27 kg/m$^2$ or more who have not been able to improve using a comprehensive lifestyle program, it is suggested that they be evaluated for potential antiobesity pharmacologic interventions. Finally, those patients with a BMI of 35 kg/m$^2$ or higher and who have not responded to the previous 2 interventions may require evaluation for bariatric surgery.

A systematic review and meta-analysis of 21 studies suggested that higher levels of alcohol consumption increased the risk of sleep apnea by 25% (risk ratio, 1.25; 95% CI, 1.13–1.38; $P<.00001$).[75] No studies were found that analyzed the impact of decreasing or eliminating alcohol consumption on OSA.

### Positive Airway Pressure

Positive airway pressure is the gold standard therapy for patients with diagnosed OSA independent of severity. Pressure to the airway is delivered through the nose or mouth with a mask. This pressure prevents the inspiratory collapse of the airway and improvement is correlated with compliance of wearing the device.[39] In a study of 2060 patients with moderate to severe OSA who were followed for an average of 8.5 years, those in the median use of continuous positive airway pressure group (6.4 h/d), decreased their risk of nonfatal and fatal cardiovascular disease events (hazard ratio [HR], 0.64; 95% CI, 0.5–0.8; $P<.001$).[76]

In another study focused on patients with OSA and atrial fibrillation, researchers noted a decrease in paroxysmal atrial fibrillation (median [IQR] 351 [2049] to 57 [182]; P = .002) and ventricular ectopy counts per 24-hour period (median [IQR] 68 [105] to 16 [133]; P = .01) at 3 months compared with baseline. Atrial ectopy at 6 months (median [IQR] 351 [2049] to 31 [113]; P = .016) was also significantly decreased. In patients with permanent atrial fibrillation at 3 months, there was also a significant reduction in ventricular ectopy (median [IQR] 100 [1116] to 33 [418]; P = .02).[77] Deng and colleagues[78] analyzed the relationship between the use of continuous positive airway pressure in patients with recurrent risk of atrial fibrillation after undergoing a catheter ablation. This meta-analysis of 10 studies included 1217 patients of whom 408 (33.52%) experienced a recurrence of atrial fibrillation after catheter ablation. Those who received continuous positive airway pressure had a lower atrial fibrillation recurrence rate than those who did not use continuous positive airway pressure (24.88% vs 42.7%; risk ratio, 0.60; 95% CI, 0.51–0.70; P = .000).

In a meta-analysis of stroke patients, with an overall adherence of 4.5 hours a night, demonstrated an overall neurofunctional improvement with use of the continuous positive airway pressure (standard mean difference, 0.5406; 95% CI, 0.0263–1.0548) based on the combined scores of the NIH Stroke Scale and Canadian Neurologic Scale.[79] Although no studies analyzed pure adherence to using the continuous positive airway pressure alone, it can be theorized that the consistent use of continuous positive airway pressure contributed to the neurologic improvements.

## Surgical

There several types of surgical procedures available for selected patients with OSA, those who have not responded to behavioral changes, and those who had difficulty using positive airway pressure devices. The surgeries include, uvulopalatopharyngoplasties, maxillomandibular advancement, and hypoglossal nerve stimulation.

### Uvulopalatopharyngoplasty

A systematic review and meta-analysis of 11 studies was completed to determine the long-term efficacy of uvulopalatopharyngoplasty.[80] Outcomes showed a significant decrease (15.4 events/h, 46.1%) in the AHI events; however, when compared with short-term outcomes (<1 year) the long-term outcomes were less effective with AHI events increasing (12.3 events/h in 63.8%). Despite the changes in surgical efficacy over time, uvulopalatopharyngoplasty remains an effective surgical method for relieving symptoms of OSA.

### Maxillomandibular Advancement

A meta-analysis of maxillomandibular advancement evaluated 45 studies with 518 different patients showing marked improvement in AHI, RDI, oxygen saturation, and surgical cure.[81] Evaluating presurgical to postsurgical AHI events, 98.8% of patients showed a significant decrease of an AHI of 20 or more events per hour (from 96.5% to 13.2%) or 30 or more events per hour (from 86.6% to 5.7%; both P<.001). Additionally, an RDI of 20 or more desaturations per hour (from 97.1% to 43.4%) and 30 or more desaturations per hour (from 91.2% to 26.5%; both P<.001). Changes in the mean ± standard deviation oxygen saturation were significant (from 70.1% ± 15.6% to 87% ± 5.2%; P<.001). Surgical cure (a decrease in events of <5 per hour) was reported in 38.5% of AHI patients and 19.1% of RDI patients, and surgical success (<20 events per hour and a decrease of ≥50% in either the AHI or the RDI) was reported in 85.5% of AHI patients and 67.6% of RDI patients. These results show that maxillomandibular advancement is a highly effective treatment for OSA; therefore, these patients do not tend to need to be hospitalized or admitted to critical care units.

### Hypoglossal Nerve Stimulation

A systematic review and meta-analysis of 12 studies with 350 patients, evaluated hypoglossal nerve stimulation clinical outcomes for patients with moderate to severe sleep apnea.[82] The AHI decrease was significant (P<.001) at 12 months with all 3 stimulators: 56.2% (Inspire), 53.5% (ImThera), and 44.3% (Apnex). At 60 months, the Inspire continued with a significant decrease in AHI events at 59.2%. The surgical success rate was 72.4% (Inspire), 76.9% (ImThera), and 55% (Apnex) also at 12 months, and at 60 months was 75% for Inspire. In the long term, there were no serious adverse events, showing that hypoglossal nerve stimulation is safe and effective for treating patients with OSA.

## INTENSIVE CARE UNIT PEARLS

Few studies focused on the care of the patient with OSA in the ICU; however, some studies provided interventions that could be applied to the care of the critically ill patient. Certain situations such as pain control, postsurgical complications, cardiac complications or desaturations, use of CPAP in the ICU continuous positive airway pressure, airway management, costs, and COVID-19 management are critical components in ICU care and with the added comorbidity of OSA require additional knowledge to provide patient-centered care.

## Pain Control

Many ICU patients experience pain during their stay requiring strong pain medications. The administration of narcotics should be considered carefully in the subset of ICU patients who also have OSA. In a study of 56 ICU patients who had PSG the night after extubation, 40 (71%) experienced sleep apnea (AHI of $\geq$5).[83] This finding was correlated with morphine given within the last 24 hours before extubation and predicted respiratory events during sleep (r = 0.35, P = .01) and sleep apnea (OR, 1.17; 95% CI, 1.02–1.34). Researchers suggested that giving high doses of opioid medications within 24 hours of extubation increased the potential for sleep apnea.

## Postoperative Complications

Patients recovering from surgery who also have OSA are at an increased risk for complications. A study of 400 patients who underwent elective musculoskeletal or abdominal surgery were analyzed for the prevalence of perioperative complications comparing those with OSA to those without.[84] Complications included more cardiovascular events (61.5% vs 8.0%; P<.0001) in the OSA group, more adverse respiratory events (13.5% vs 3.2%; P<.0001), more urinary tract infections (4.2% vs 0%; P<.0001), more difficult intubations (2.5% vs 0.2%; P<.01), and more prolonged awakening from anesthesia (2.5% vs 0%; P<.001).

## Cardiac Complications and Desaturation

In a prospective cohort study, 1218 patients were analyzed for 30-day cardiovascular complications (myocardial injury, cardiac death, heart failure, thromboembolism, atrial fibrillation, and stroke) after undergoing major noncardiac surgery.[85] Of patients with severe OSA, 30.1% (41/136), 22.1% (52/235) with moderate OSA, 19.0% (86/452) with mild OSA, and 14.2% (56/395) with no OSA, developed cardiovascular complications 30 days after surgery. The was an association between OSA and a higher risk of developing cardiovascular complications (adjusted HR, 149 [95% CI, 1.19–2.01]; P = .1); however, the association was only significant in patients with severe OSA (adjusted HR, 2.23 [95% CI, 1.49–3.34] P = .001). Additionally, the mean cumulative duration of oxyhemoglobin desaturation of 80% or lower during the first 3 nights postoperatively in patients with cardiovascular complications (23.1 minutes [95% CI, 15.5–27.7 minutes]) was longer than in those without (10.2 minutes [95% CI, 7.8–10.9 minutes]; P<.001). Additional post hoc analyses determined that OSA was associated with myocardial injury (adjusted HR, 1.80 [95% CI, 1.17–2.77]), atrial fibrillation (adjusted HR, 3.96 [95% CI, 1.24–12.60]), congestive heart failure (adjusted HR, 6.55 [95% CI, 1.71–25.06]), and cardiac death (adjusted HR, 13.66 [95% CI, 1.63–114.19]). Each of these events were associated with oxygen saturation levels of less than 80%. The application of this information might suggest that interventions to prevent desaturation in cardiac patients with known OSA should be investigated further. In a randomized, double-blind, single-center trial, 106 patients with a medium to high risk for OSA underwent an elective surgery.[86] The transcutaneous electrical stimulus group (n = 34) has a stimulus applied when oxygen saturation measurements reached 93% or less. It was noted that a lower percentage of patients in the transcutaneous electrical stimulus group registered an $SpO_2$ of less than 90 (47% vs 71%; $P = .03$), a shorter duration of time with an of $SpO_2$ less than 90 (median 0.0 seconds vs 19.1 seconds $P = .01$), and a higher nadir of $SpO_2$ recorded during the first hour (median 90.5% vs 87.9%; $P = .04$). Although this was a single-center trial and needs replication, the research suggests that transcutaneous electrical stimulus may decrease the duration and magnitude of hypoxemia.

### Continuous Positive Airway Pressure in the Intensive Care Unit

Patient outcomes improve with the consistent wearing of positive airway pressure/ continuous positive airway pressure devices and this practice should be continued for the OSA patient during their ICU stay.[87] In a randomized controlled parallel group study, the association of the use of continuous positive airway pressure with metabolic events was analyzed. Twenty-six patients underwent PSG nightly in the laboratory for 2 weeks and glucose metabolism was assessed at baseline and after 2 weeks with both oral and IV glucose tolerance tests. Researchers found that the overall glucose response was reduced (treatment difference, $-1276.9$ [mg/dL] min [95% CI, $-2,392.4$ to -161.5]; $P = .03$) and insulin sensitivity was improved (treatment difference: 0.77 $[mU/L]^{-1}$ $min^{-1}$ [95% CI, 0.03–1.52]; $P = .04$) with continuous positive airway pressure. Additionally, norepinephrine levels were significantly lower (treatment difference, $-111.4$; 95% CI, $-175.5$ to $-47.4$; $P = .001$), 24-hour systolic blood pressure (treatment difference, $-9.5$ [95% CI, $-16.6$ to $-2.4$]; $P = .009$), daytime systolic blood pressure (treatment difference, $-9.7$ [95% CI, $-16.8$ to $- 2.5$]; $P = .008$), nighttime systolic blood pressure (treatment difference, $-10.8$ [95% CI, $-20.7$ to $-0.8$]; $P = .04$), 24-hour diastolic blood pressure (treatment difference, $-7.1$ [95% CI, $-10.9$ to $-3.2$]; $P<.001$); day time diastolic blood pressure (treatment difference, $-8.2$ [95% CI, $-12.5$ to $-3.9$; $P<.001$), and nighttime diastolic blood pressure (treatment difference, $-6.1$ [95% CI, $-11.4$ to $-0.8$]; $P = .02$). This study was not conducted in an ICU, but the results could still be applied to critically ill patients.

### Airway Management

Evidence from a meta-analysis determined that patients with OSA are at an increased risk for difficult intubation, which may be in part due to anatomic changes in the airway, neck circumference, and obesity.[88] Patients with OSA experienced more difficult intubations, difficult mask ventilation, and failed supraglottic airway insertions. Overall, the odds for a difficult intubation were increased for patients with OSA versus patients without OSA (13.5% vs 2.5%; pooled OR, 3.46; 95% CI, 2.32–5.16, $P<.00001$). Difficult mask ventilation was significantly higher in patients with OSA when compared with patients without OSA (4.48% vs 1.11%; pooled OR, 3.39; 95% CI, 2.74–4.18, $P<.00001$). There were several failed supraglottic airway insertions; however, there was no statistically significant difference between those with or without OSA. Understanding that patients with OSA are at a higher risk for airway management issues will allow health care professionals to be prepared to provide potential preventative care to mitigate airway issues.

### Cost

Patients who spend more time in the ICU tend to generate more costs. In a retrospective study of 5146 patients with 289 who had OSA, there was no impact of OSA on ICU mortality, in-hospital mortality, or ventilator-associated pneumonia; however, ICU length of stay was statistically significantly longer for the patient who had OSA and a BMI of more than 40 kg/m$^2$ (incident rate ratio, 1.56; 95% CI, 1.05–2.32; $P = .03$).[89]

## Coronavirus Disease-2019

As ICUs continue to admit patients with COVID-19, it will be necessary to determine if patients with OSA require specific interventions. In 1 study, OSA was noted to be independently associated with increased risk of death on day 7 of COVID-19 (OR, 2.90; 95% CI, 1.46–5.38).[90] In another study, OSA was noted to have common risk factors and comorbidities with patients who have poor COVID-19 outcomes. This finding suggests that patients with OSA may be at an increased risk of death from COVID-19.[91]

## SUMMARY

Individuals with OSA may never need care in a critical care unit; however, when they do the team must be prepared to provide interventions that will enhance patient outcomes. There is a significant gap in the literature regarding specific interventions the critical care nurse should implement to care for patients diagnosed with OSA. This may be in part to the significant unrecognition of OSA, which then impacts the number of patients diagnosed with OSA. Providing education to critical care practitioners regarding clinical presentation and diagnoses enhances knowledge and awareness to assess for OSA in the critical care population and provide cares, which decrease complications, improve sleep, and enhance patient outcomes. Although specific interventions still need to be researched, critical care practitioners can recognize that much of the care they are already providing can positively impact a patient with OSA.

Critically ill patients often experience pain during their stay in the ICU and nurses provide opioids to minimize their pain. Research has shown that high doses of opioids are correlated with an increased risk for sleep apnea.[83] The critical care nurse aware of this information can seek alternative methods of providing pain management for critically ill patients.

Armed with knowledge, the critical care nurse will be aware that patients with OSA are more likely to have adverse cardiac and respiratory events, as well as urinary tract infections, and are more difficult to intubate and wake up more slowly from anesthesia.[85,88] Patients with OSA can be monitored with additional care taken to prevent these complications common with a variety of diagnoses. Critical care nurses are trained to be acutely aware of oxygen saturation levels. Knowing that hypoxemic events are more likely to trigger both respiratory and cardiac complications in patients with OSA, the nurse knows to intervene more quickly to maintain appropriate oxygen saturation levels.[84,85,87] Knowing that patients who have difficult or failed intubation attempts or for whom ventilation via mask is a struggle, often have OSA can alert the critical care team to further analyze and potentially diagnose the patient with previously unrecognized OSA.[88]

Several studies spoke to the importance of continuous positive airway pressure in mitigating complications of OSA.[39,76–79,87] The critical care nurse should advocate for the use of continuous positive airway pressure for patients with OSA during their hospitalization. This practice will not impact those with undiagnosed OSA; however, for patients who are alert and oriented, implementing the use of the STOP-BANG Questionnaire to determine the potential for underlying OSA allows for potential recognition of OSA and thus further treatment.

As more patients are being admitted to critical care units with COVID-19, it is imperative to understand to the potential correlation with OSA. Critical care nurses need to be aware of this correlation and question family members regarding a history of OSA or if they have noted any signs and symptoms of OSA that may indicate the patient already has OSA.[91] Early treatment will allow for early intervention, which can enhance patient outcomes.

Last, as critical care practitioners examine budgetary issues and recognize that some length of stay costs may be attributable to patients with OSA, it becomes crucial to conduct further studies to identify unrecognized OSA in the critical care setting and develop of specific interventions to decrease cost and positively impact patient outcomes.[89] As patients become increasingly complex and more diverse in terms of their needs, it is important for critical care practitioners to meet this challenge with an interprofessional approach to provide high-quality critical care.

## CLINICS CARE POINTS

---

- It is important to recognize that all hospitalized patients are likely experiencing sleep deprivation.
- Closely monitor OSA patients when administering analgesics particularly those who have been recently extubated or during sleep as these are high risk periods.
- OSA patients are at a higher risk for adverse cardiovascular and respiratory events, experience more UTIs, are more difficult to intubation and take longer to wake up after receiving anesthesia.
- Maintaining oxygen saturation is important for all patients but patients with OSA are more likely to experience deleterious impacts from low levels.
- OSA patients who utilize CPAP at home should continue to use CPAP while hospitalized.

---

## DISCLOSURE

The author has nothing to disclose.

## REFERENCES

1. Hafner M, Stepanek M, Taylor J, et al. Why sleep matters-the economic cost of insufficient sleep. Rand Health Q 2017;6(4):11. Available at: https://www.ncbi.nlm.nih.gov/pmc/articles/PMC5627640/#!po=85.8974.
2. Grimm J. Sleep deprivation in the intensive care patient. Crit Care Nurse 2020;40(2):e16–24.
3. Garvey JF, Pengo MF, Drakatos P, et al. Epidemiological aspects of obstructive sleep apnea. J Thorac Dis 2015;7(5):920–9.
4. Asif N, Iqbal R, Nazier CF. Review Article Human immune system during sleep. Am J Clin Exp Immunol 2017;6(6):92–6. Available at: https://www.ncbi.nlm.nih.gov/pmc/articles/PMC5768894/pdf/ajcei0006-0092.pdf.
5. Tan HL, Kheirandish-Gozal L, Gozal D. Sleep, sleep disorders, and immune function. In: Fishbein A, Sheldon SH, editors. Allergy in sleep. Switzerland: Springer Nature; 2019. p. 3–15. Available at: https://www.researchgate.net/publication/334088440_Pharmacologic_Management_of_Allergic_Disease_and_Sleep.
6. Fleming WE, Ferouz-Colborn A, Samoszuk MK, et al. Blood biomarkers of endocrine, immune, inflammatory, and metabolic systems in obstructive sleep apnea. Clin Biochem 2016;49(12):854–61.
7. Wright KP, Drake AL, Frey DL, et al. Influence of sleep deprivation and circadian misalignment on cortisol, inflammatory markers, and cytokine balance. Brain Behav Immun 2015;47:24–34.

8. During EH, Kawai M. The functions of sleep and the effects of sleep deprivation. In: Miglis M, editor. Sleep and neurologic disease. Academic Press; 2017. p. 55–72. Available at: https://www.sciencedirect.com/science/article/pii/B9780128040744000030.

9. Al-Abari MA, Jaju D, Al-Sinani S, et al. Habitual sleep deprivation is associated with type 2 diabetes: a case-control study. Oman Med J 2016;31(6):399–403.

10. Ryan S. Adipose tissue inflammation by intermittent hypoxia: mechanistic link between obstructive sleep apnoea and metabolic dysfunction. J Physiol 2017; 585(8):2423–30.

11. Huang R, Lin BM, Stampfer MJ, et al. A population-based study of the bidirectional association between obstructive sleep apnea and type 2 diabetes in three prospective U.S. cohorts. Diabetes Care 2018;41:2111–9.

12. Dres M, Youness M, Rittayamai N, et al. Sleep and pathological wakefulness at time of liberation from mechanical ventilation (SLEEWE): a prospective multicenter physiological study. Am J Respir Crit Med 2019;199(9):1106–15.

13. Rault C, Sangare A, Diaz V, et al. The impact of sleep deprivation on respiratory motor output and endurance A Physiological Study. Am J Respir Crit Med 2020; 201(8):976–83.

14. Maas MB, Kim M, Malkani RG, et al. Obstructive sleep apnea and risk of COVID-19 infection, hospitalization and respiratory failure. Sleep Breath 2020. https://doi.org/10.1007/s11325-020-02203-0.

15. Lowe CJ, Safati A, Hall PA. The neurocognitive consequences of sleep restriction: a meta-analytic review. Neurosci Biobehavioral Rev 2017;80(2017):586–604.

16. Phua CS, Jayaram L, Wijeratne T. Relationship between sleep duration and risk factors for stroke. Front Neurol 2017;8(392). https://doi.org/10.3389/fneur.2017.00392.

17. Jehan S, Farag M, Zizi F, et al. Obstructive sleep apnea and stroke. Sleep Med Disord 2018;2(5):120–5. Available at: https://www.ncbi.nlm.nih.gov/pmc/articles/PMC6340906/pdf/nihms-1004011.pdf.

18. Dong R, Dong Z, Liu H, et al. Prevalence, risk factors, outcomes, and treatment of obstructive sleep apnea in patients with cerebrovascular disease: a systematic review. J Stroke Cerebrovasc Dis 2018;27(6):1471–80.

19. Kohansieh M, Makaryus AN. Sleep deficiency and deprivation leading to cardiovascular disease. Int J Hypertens 2015;2015. https://doi.org/10.1155/2015/615681.

20. Liu H, Chen A. Roles of sleep deprivation in cardiovascular dysfunctions. Life Sci 2019;219:231–7.

21. Aurora RN, Crainiceanu C, Gottlieb DJ, et al. Obstructive sleep apnea during REM sleep and cardiovascular disease. Am J Respir Crit Med 2018;197(5):653–60.

22. Jehan S, Zizi F, Pandi-Perumal SR, et al. Obstructive sleep apnea and obesity: implications for public health. Sleep Med Disord 2017;1(4). Available at: https://www.ncbi.nlm.nih.gov/pmc/articles/PMC5836788/pdf/nihms932293.pdf.

23. Peppard PE, Young T, Palta M. Longitudinal study of moderate weight change and sleep-disordered breathing. JAMA 2000;284(23):3015–21.

24. Lin H, Xiong H, Ji C, et al. Upper airway lengthening caused by weight increase in obstructive sleep apnea patients. Respir Res 2020;21(272). https://doi.org/10.1186/s12931-020-01532-8.

25. Mukherjee S, Patel SR, Kales SN, et al. An official American thoracic society statement: the importance of health sleep. Am J Respir Crit Med 2015;191(12):1450–8.

26. Leary EB, Watson KT, Ancoli-Israel S, et al. Association of rapid eye movement sleep with mortality in middle-aged and older adults. JAMA Neurol 2020; 77(10):1241–51.

27. Reznik ME, Slooter AJC. Delirium management in the ICU. Curr Treat Options Neurol 2019;21(59). https://doi.org/10.1007/s11940-019-0599-5.

28. Evans JL, Nadler JW, Preud'homme XA, et al. Pilot prospective study of post-surgical sleep and EEG predictors of post-operative delirium. Clin Neurophysiol 2017;128(2017):1421–5.

29. Salluh JIF, Wang H, Schneider EB, et al. Outcome of delirium in critically ill patients: systematic review and meta-analysis. BMJ 2015;(h2538):350. https://doi.org/10.1136/gmj.h2538.

30. Senaratna CV, Perret JL, Lodge CJ, et al. Prevalence of obstructive sleep apnea in the general population: a systematic review. Sleep Med Rev 2017;34:70–81.

31. Bauters FA, Hertegonne KB, De Buyzere ML, et al. Phenotype and risk burden of sleep apnea: a population-based cohort study. Hypertension 2019;74:1052–62.

32. Johnson DA, Guo N, Rueschman M, et al. Prevalence and correlates of obstructive sleep apnea among African-Americans: the Jackson heart sleep study. SleepJ 2018;1–9. https://doi.org/10.1093/sleep/zsy154.

33. Jackson M, Becerra BJ, Marmolejo C, et al. Prevalence and correlates of sleep apnea among US male veterans, 2005 – 2014. Prev Chronic Dis 2017;14:160365.

34. Tveit RL, Lehmann S, Bjorvatn B. Prevalence of several somatic diseases depends on the presence and severity of obstructive sleep apnea. PLoS One 2018;13(2):e0192671.

35. Bailly S, Galerneau LM, Ruckly S, et al. Impact of obstructive sleep apnea on the obesity paradox in critically ill patients. Journal of Critical Care 2020;56:120–4. https://doi.org/10.1016/j.jcrc.2019.12.016.

36. Bolona E, Hahn PY, Afessa B. Intensive care unit and hospital mortality in patients with obstructive sleep apnea. J Crit Care 2015;30(1):178–80.

37. Jean RE, Gibson CD, Jean RA, et al. Obstructive sleep apnea and acute respiratory failure: an analysis of mortality risk in patients with pneumonia requiring mechanical ventilation. J Crit Care 2015;30(2015):778–83.

38. Franklin KA, Lindberg E. Obstructive sleep apnea is a common disorder in the population – a review on the epidemiology of sleep apnea. J Thorac Dis 2015; 7(8):1311–22.

39. Gottlieb DJ, Punjabi NM. Diagnosis and management of obstructive sleep apnea: a review. JAMA 2020;323(14):1389–400.

40. Spector AR, Loriaux D, Farjat AE. The clinical significance of apneas versus hypopneas: is there really a difference? Cureus 2019;11(4):e4560.

41. Zinchuk A, Gentry M, Concato J, et al. Phenotypes in obstructive sleep apnea: a definition, examples and evolution of approaches. Sleep Med Rev 2017;35: 113–23.

42. Destors M, Tamisier R, Galerneau LM, et al. Pathophysiology of obstructive sleep apnea-hypopnea syndrome and its cardiometabolic consequences. Article in French. Presse Med 2017;46(4):395–403.

43. Mehra R. Sleep apnea and the heart. Cleve Clin J Med 2019;86(suppl 1):10–8.

44. White LH, Bradley TD. Role of nocturnal rostral fluid shift in the pathogenesis of obstructive and central sleep apnoea. J Physiol 2013;591(5):1179–93.

45. Veasey SC, Rosen IM. Obstructive sleep apnea in adults. N Engl J Med 2019; 380:1442–9.

46. Semelka M, Wilson J, Floyd R. Diagnosis and treatment of obstructive sleep apnea in adults. Am Fam Physician 2016;94(5):355–60. Available at: https://www.aafp.org/afp/2016/0901/afp20160901p355.pdf.

47. Arnold J, Sunilkumar M, Krishna V, et al. Obstructive sleep apnea. J Pharm Bioallied Sci 2017;9(suppl 1):S26–8.

48. Laratta CR, Ayas NT, Povitz M, et al. Diagnosis and treatment of obstructive sleep apnea in adults. CMAJ 2017;189(48):e1481–8.

49. Miller JN, Berger AM. Screening and assessment for obstructive sleep apnea in primary care. Sleep Med Rev 2016;29(2016):41–51.

50. Perger E, Badarani O, Philippe C, et al. Evening sock marks as an adjunct to the clinical prediction of obstructive sleep apnea. Sleep Breath 2020;24(4):1365–71.

51. Spalka J, Kedzia K, Kuczynski W, et al. Morning headache as an obstructive sleep apnea-related symptom among sleep clinic patients-a cross-section analysis. Brain Sci 2020;10(57). https://doi.org/10.3390/brainsci10010057.

52. Ljunggren M, Lindberg D, Franklin KA, et al. Obstructive sleep apnea during rapid eye movement sleep is associated with early signs of atherosclerosis in women. Sleep 2018;41(7). https://doi.org/10.1093/sleep/zsy099.

53. Korkalainen H, Toyras J, Nikkonen S, et al. Mortality-risk-based apnea-hypopnea index thresholds for diagnostics of obstructive sleep apnea. J Sleep Res 2019;28:e12855–63.

54. Punjabi NM. Is the apnea-hypopnea index the best way to quantify the severity of sleep-disordered breathing? No Chest 2016;149(1):16–9.

55. Ho V, Crainiceanu CM, Punjabi NM, et al. Calibration model for apnea-hypopnea indices: impact of alternative criteria for hypopneas. Sleep 2015;38(12):1887–92.

56. Rundo JW, Downey R. Polysomnography. In: Levin KH, Chauvel P, editors. Handbook of clinical Neurology, vol. 160. Elsevier; 2019. p. 381–91. https://doi.org/10.1016/B7978-0-444-64032-1.00025-4.

57. Malhotra RK, Kirsch DB, Kristo DA, et al. Polysomnography for obstructive sleep apnea should include arousal-based scoring: an American academy of sleep medicine position statement. J Clin Sleep Med 2018;14(7):1245–7.

58. AASM clarifies hypopnea scoring criteria. American Academy of Sleep Medicine. 2013. Available at: https://aasm.org/aasm-clarifies-hypopnea-scoring-criteria/. Accessed December 24, 2020.

59. Kapur VK, Donovan LM. Why a single index to measure sleep apnea is not enough. J Clin Sleep Med 2019;15(5):867–96.

60. Trevethan R. Sensitivity, specificity, and predictive values: foundations, pliabilities, and pitfalls in research and practice. Front Public Health 2017;5(307). https://doi.org/10.3389/fpubh.2017.00307.

61. Nagappa M, Wong J, Singh M, et al. An update on the various practical applications of the STOP-Bang questionnaire in anesthesia, surgery, and perioperative medicine. Curr Opin Anesthesiol 2017;30:118–215.

62. Popevic MB, Milovanovic A, Nagorni-Obradovia L, et al. Screening commercial drivers for obstructive sleep apnea: validation of stop-bang questionnaire. Int J Occup Med Environ Health 2017;30(5):751–61.

63. Abumuamar AA, Dorian P, Newman D, et al. The STOP-BANG questionnaire shows an insufficient specificity for detecting obstructive sleep apnea in patients with atrial fibrillation. J Sleep Res 2018;27:e12702.

64. Prasad KT, Sehgal IS, Agarwal R, et al. Assessing the likelihood of obstructive sleep apnea: a comparison of nine screening questionnaires. Sleep Breath 2017;24(4):909–17.

65. Lapin BR, Bena JF, Walia HK, et al. The Epworth sleepiness scale: validation of one-dimensional factor structure in a large clinical Sample. J Clin Sleep Med 2019;14(8):1293–301.

66. Senaratna CV, Perret JL, Lowe A, et al. Detecting sleep apnoea syndrome in primary care with screening questionnaires and the Epworth sleepiness scale. MJA 2019;211(2):65–70.

67. Guo Q, Song Wd, Li Wei, et al. Weighted Epworth sleepiness scale predicted the apnea-hypopnea index better. Respir Res 2020;21(147). https://doi.org/10.1186/s12931-020-01417-w.

68. Khaledi-Paveh B, Khazaie H, Nasouri M, et al. Evaluation of Berlin questionnaire validity for sleep apnea risk in sleep clinic populations. Basic Clin Neurosci 2016; 7(1):43–8. Available at: https://www.ncbi.nlm.nih.gov/pmc/articles/PMC4892329/pdf/BCN-7-43.pdf.

69. Ng SS, Tam W, Chan TO, et al. Use of Berlin questionnaire in comparison to polysomnography and home sleep study in patients with obstructive sleep apnea. Respir Res 2019;20(40). https://doi.org/10.1186/s12931-019-1009-y.

70. Tan A, Yim JD, Tan LW, et al. Using the Berlin questionnaire to predict obstructive sleep apnea in the general population. J Clin Sleep Med 2017;13(3):427–32.

71. Wu Q, Xie L, Li W, et al. Pulmonary function influences the performance of Berlin questionnaire, modified Berlin questionnaire, and STOP-bang score for screening obstructive sleep apnea in subjects with chronic obstructive pulmonary disease. Int J Chron Obstruct Pulmon Dis 2020;15:1207–16.

72. Armon C. Polysomnography: overview, parameters monitored, staging of sleep. Medscape 2020. Available at: https://emedicine.medscape.com/article/1188764-overview#a1.

73. Igelstrom H, Asenlof P, Emtner M, et al. Improvement in obstructive sleep apnea after a tailored behavioural sleep medicine intervention targeting healthy eating and physical activity: a randomized controlled trial. Sleep Breath 2018;22: 653–61.

74. Hudgel DW, Patel SR, Ihasic AM, et al. The role of weight management in the treatment of adult obstructive sleep apnea: an official American Thoracic Society clinical practice guideline. Am J Respir Crit Care Med 2018;198(6):e70–8.

75. Simou E, Britton J, Leonardi-Bee J. Alcohol and the risk of sleep apnoea: a systematic review and meta-analysis. Sleep Med 2018;42:38–46.

76. Myllyla M, Hammais A, Stepanov M, et al. Nonfatal and fatal cardiovascular disease events in CPAP compliant obstructive sleep apnea patients. Sleep Breath 2019;23:1209–17.

77. Abumuamar AA, Newman D, Dorian P, et al. Cardiac effects of CPAP treatment in patients with obstructive sleep apnea and atrial fibrillation. J Interv Card Electrophysiol 2019;54:289–97.

78. Deng F, Raza A, Guo J. Treating obstructive sleep apnea with continuous positive airway pressure reduces risk of recurrent atrial fibrillation after catheter ablation: a meta-analysis. Sleep Med 2018;46:5–11.

79. Brill AK, Horvth T, Seiler A, et al. CPAP as treatment of sleep apnea after stroke. Neurology 2018;90:21222.e30.

80. He M, Yin F, Zhan S, et al. Long-term efficacy of uvulopalatrpharyngoplasty among adult patients with obstructive sleep apnea: a systematic review and meta-analysis. Otolaryngol Head Neck Surg 2019;161(3):401–11.

81. Zaghi S, Holty JEC, Certal V, et al. Maxillomandibular advancement for treatment of obstructive sleep apnea: a meta-analysis. JAMA Otolaryngol Head Neck Surg 2016;142(1):58–66.

82. Costantino A, Rinaldi V, Moffa A, et al. Hypoglossal nerve stimulation long-term clinical outcomes: a systematic review and meta-analysis. Sleep Breath 2020; 24(2):399–411.
83. Timm FP, Zaremba S, Grabitz SD, et al. Effects of opioids given to facilitate mechanical ventilation on sleep apnea after extubation in the intensive care unit. Sleep 2018;41(1). https://doi.org/10.1093/sleep/zsx191.
84. Ambrosii T, Sandru S, Belii A. The prevalence of perioperative complications in patients with and without obstructive sleep apnoea: a prospective cohort study. Rom J Anaesth Intensive Care 2016;23(2):103–10.
85. Chan MTV, Wang CY, Seet E, et al. Association of unrecognized obstructive sleep apnea with postoperative cardiovascular events in patients undergoing major noncardiac surgery. JAMA 2019;321(18):1788–98.
86. Smith HM, Kilger J, Burkle CM, et al. Peripheral electrical stimulation reduces postoperative hypoxemia in patients at risk for obstructive sleep apnea: a randomized-controlled trial. Can J Anesth 2019;66:1296–309.
87. Padmidi S, Wroblewski K, Stepien M, et al. Eight hours of nightly continuous positive airway pressure treatment of obstructive sleep apnea improves glucose metabolism in patients with prediabetes: a randomized controlled trial. AM J Respir Crit Care Med 2015;192(1):96–105.
88. Nagappa M, Wong DT, Cozowicz C, et al. Is obstructive sleep apnea associated with difficult airway? Evidence from a systematic review and meta-analysis of prospective and retrospective cohort studies. PLoS One 2018;13(10):e0204904.
89. Bailly S, Galerneau LM, Ruckly S, et al. Impact of obstructive sleep apnea on the obesity paradox in critically ill patients. J Crit Care 2020;56:120–4.
90. Cariou B, Hadjadj S, Wargny M, et al. Phenotypic characteristics and prognosis of inpatients with COVID-19 and diabetes: the CORONADO study. Diabetologia 2020;63:1500–15.
91. Miller MA, Cappuccio FP. A systematic review of COVID-19 and obstructive sleep apnoea. Sleep Med Rev 2021;55:101382.

# Benefits of Early Mobility on Sleep in the Intensive Care Unit

Jaime Rohr, MSN, RN-BC*

## KEYWORDS

- Early mobility • Rehabilitation • Sleep • Intensive care unit
- Mobility barriers/solutions

## KEY POINTS

- Early mobility improves patient sleep in the intensive care unit.
- Patient participation in exercise activities prevents further complications.
- Nurses should incorporate mobility interventions daily.
- Strategies to overcome mobility barriers should be an interdisciplinary approach.
- Personalized mobility plans allow for safe implementation.

## INTRODUCTION

Early patient mobility in the intensive care unit (ICU) has numerous benefits. Improved sleep and prevention of complications are known benefits of incorporating early mobility into the ICU patient's plan of care. Despite the known benefits of early mobilization, the complex nature of the ICU patient conditions can create barriers to its use. Nurses can use the ABCDEF bundle (**Table 1**) to help prioritize and organize their care to include mobility with other life-saving interventions. Keeping in mind the importance of sleep in the ICU patient, and knowing that early mobility improves sleep, nurses can better understand the importance of incorporating mobility into daily care.

## REVIEW OF LITERATURE
### Early Mobility

Nurses often provide care by the adage, rehabilitation begins at admission. Early mobility of the ICU patient is one component of rehabilitation. Zhang and associates[1] evaluated 13 studies and summarized that early mobility is initiated within 5 days of admission. Early mobility has been shown to prevent complications and expedites the return to premorbid status.[2] Benefits of early ICU mobility include increased

Bronson School of Nursing, Western Michigan University, Kalamazoo, MI, USA
* 56221 Fairway Drive, Paw Paw, MI.
E-mail address: jaime.rohr@wmich.edu

Crit Care Nurs Clin N Am 33 (2021) 193–201
https://doi.org/10.1016/j.cnc.2021.01.007
0899-5885/21/© 2021 Elsevier Inc. All rights reserved.

**Table 1**
**ABCDEF definition**

| | |
|---|---|
| A = | Assessing, preventing, and managing pain |
| B = | Breathing trials and spontaneous awakening |
| C = | Choice analgesia and sedation |
| D = | Delirium assessment, prevention, and management |
| E = | Early mobility |
| F = | Family engagement and empowerment |

*Data adapted from* Schallom and colleagues Implementation of an interdisciplinary AACN early mobility protocol. *Critical Care Nurse,* 2020;40(4):7 to 17.

sleep quality, reduced ventilator days, shortened length of hospitalization, prevention of numerous complications, and improved functional outcomes.[3] Common complications from lack of patient mobility include sleep alterations, pneumonia, pressure ulcers, deep vein thrombosis, urinary tract infection, loss of muscle mass, ICU-acquired weakness, increased length of hospital stay, increased morbidity, and mortality.[4-7] Sleep is identified as a modifiable patient risk factor.[8] Exercise is one intervention that helps improve sleep and change this risk factor for patients in the ICU.

National organizations involved with critical care view increasing patient mobility in the ICU as a priority.[9] Early patient mobility is part of a set of evidence-based practices known as the ABCDEF bundle (refer to **Table 1**). This bundle is a set of clinical practice standards to improve patient outcomes in the critically ill. Outcomes improved with this bundle include a shortened length of stay, increased survival, reduced days requiring mechanical ventilation, less delirium, more restraint-free care, and lower ICU readmission rates.[9-11] Early mobilization has been identified as the most effective nonpharmacologic intervention to reduce delirium.[12] Understanding and using the ABCDEF bundle can help nurses and other ICU staff provide quality patient care and help minimize additional complications.

### Mobility and Sleep Quality

Patient mobility levels, or lack thereof, impact sleep. Early mobilization has been found to promote sleep.[13] Quality of sleep has been shown to worsen for patients who are in bed and immobile for prolonged periods of time.[7] It is common for ICU patients to spend most of their time in bed due to the severity of their conditions. Fragmentation of sleep is a known problem for the ICU patient due to necessary care that interferes with their ability to sleep uninterrupted for long periods of time. More than half of patients in the ICU report poor sleep quality, describing it as broken, light, frequent interruptions, difficulty falling asleep, and not feeling well rested.[7,8]

Reduction in normal activity level plays a role in sleep alterations in the ICU when patients are not at their mobility baseline due to their critical illness. Immobility and restricted mobility related to lines, tubes, or catheters were identified as a common cause of sleep disruptions in critically ill individuals.[8] Mobility exercises while hospitalized can help minimize patient sleep complications. If a patient must be confined to their bed, mobility exercises can be revised to meet those restrictions and abilities. Bedrest or inability to get out of bed does not, and should not, prevent mobility-based interventions. The closer to admission patient mobility begins, the better the outcomes will be. Nurses are in a unique position at the bedside to act as advocates to make early patient mobilization in the ICU a reality.

Daytime exercise has been shown to increase sleep latency, nighttime sleep, and help maintain a healthy circadian rhythm.[14–16] It is not recommended for patients to be physically active at night or directly before bedtime.[14] Falling in and out of sleep during the daytime occurs less frequently when patients have increased activity and this promotes increased sleep at night.[15] Nurses can plan patient mobility interventions during the day to follow these recommendations. Patients in the ICU who participate in an exercise program fall asleep faster and experience increased quality of sleep compared with those with no exercise interventions. Sleep in the ICU is crucial for patient recovery, and mobility interventions can help improve its quality and promote feelings of restfulness.

### Mobility Modalities and Rehabilitation

Clinical practice guidelines suggest mobilization of critically ill adults.[8] Early patient mobility can come in many forms and should be an interdisciplinary approach, including nurses, physical therapists, occupational therapists, respiratory therapists, physicians, and all other bedside care staff.[9] To maximize patient physical effort, the interdisciplinary care team needs to focus on communication, cooperation, and personalizing the daily planning of care, goals, and interventions.[13]

Most ICU patients are unable to perform lengthy exercise but can complete shorter periods of activity. Passive movements, ambulation, and all mobility levels in between are helpful for patients in preventing complications and promoting sleep. All mobility interventions need to be personalized to patient needs and abilities. This personalized care planning is essential, as it allows for safe implementation with patient restrictions and conditions. Refer to **Box 1** for examples of mobility modalities.

Physical rehabilitation activities can have a positive impact on patient sleep quality and a combination of rehabilitation and mobilization is helpful. Patient rehabilitation consists of interventions to optimize physical functioning and limit disabilities, whereas

---

**Box 1**
**Mobility modalities**

Passive range of motion

Passive limb exercises

Repositioning

Stretching

Active range of motion

Dangling on edge of bed

Sitting in a chair

Standing

Marching in place

Ambulating in room

Ambulating in hall

*Data from*: Schallom M, Tymkew H, Vyers K, Prentice D, Sona C, Norris T, Arroyo C. (2020). Implementation of an interdisciplinary AACN early mobility protocol. *Critical Care Nurse*, 2020;40(4):7-17 and Younis G, Sayed Ahmed S. Effectiveness of passive range of motion exercise on hemodynamic parameters and behavioral pain intensity among adult mechanically ventilated patients. *IOSR Journal of Nursing and Health Science*. 2015;4(6):47-59.

mobilization is an intervention used to facilitate patient movement and range of motion.[8] Increased physical activity correlates with improved sleep quality, and decreased physical activity is linked to decreased quality of sleep.[15] Poor sleep quality results in increased daytime drowsiness, which makes energy for mobility lower, and creates a cycle of disturbed sleep patterns due to circadian rhythm alterations.[15] Position changes can be planned with bedtime care to aid in comfort and help with patient sleep.[17]

Many ICU patients are unable to complete mobility activities independently and may require assistance or passive limb exercises (PLE). Repeated movements of a joint within tolerable limits, performed without patient control, is the definition of PLEs.[18] Passive mobility is useful in preventing ICU complications and patients who are unable to complete movements independently could benefit from PLEs to meet early mobilization recommendations. Benefits of passive activities can include better sleep quality, increase in venous return, maintained joint ranges, decrease in contractures, improved pain management, and overall reduced total hospital stay.[7,8,18]

Successful mobility progression requires early patient interventions that are personalized and support mobilization. Patient mobility capabilities should improve with a rehabilitation plan and as their condition stabilizes closer to ICU discharge. Nurses and other members of the interdisciplinary team can use different mobility modalities as their patient condition tolerates. See **Box 2** for the American Association of Critical Care Nurses (AACN) mobility progression recommendations.

### Intensive Care Unit–Acquired Weakness

Intensive care unit–acquired weakness (ICUAW) results in generalized muscle weakness that can impact peripheral and respiratory muscles with no other known causes

---

**Box 2**
**Mobility progression recommendation**

Passive range of motion
↓
Active range of motion
↓
Staff repositioning
↓
Assisted turning
↓
Self-turning
↓
Sitting position
↓
Sitting on the edge of the bed
↓
Sitting in a chair
↓
Marching in place
↓
Walking in halls

Data adapted from Schallom et al. Implementation of an interdisciplinary AACN early mobility protocol. *Critical Care Nurse*, 2020;40(4):7-17.

outside of their critical illness.[6] ICUAW is a common occurrence and can be found in 25% to 50% of critically ill patients.[6,8,19] Each day of bed rest reduces muscle strength 3% to 11% and it can take weeks or even months to return to baseline strength.[20] Prolonged immobilization or bed rest is one of the risk factors along with illness severity, sepsis, multiorgan failure, and hyperglycemia.[6] Early mobility interventions can help mitigate the risk of developing ICUAW and is another reason to prioritize patient rehabilitation and mobilization with daily care.

## Barriers to Intensive Care Unit Mobility Implementation

Despite the identified benefits of early patient mobility in the ICU, staff face potential barriers to its implementation (**Box 3**). Respiratory complications and hemodynamic instability are identified as the main barriers that prevent early mobility in the ICU.[5,18] Staff may perceive vasoactive medications and mechanical ventilation as mobility barriers but in otherwise stable patients mobilization should not be

---

**Box 3**
**Potential barriers to patient mobility in the Intensive Care Unit (ICU)**

- Neurologic impairments
- Respiratory status
- Mechanical ventilation
- Hemodynamic instability
- Deep sedation
- Acuity of illness
- Patient pain level
- Delirium
- Inability to follow commands
- Communication barriers
- Limited equipment
- No mobility protocols
- Patient body weight
- Inadequate staff education
- ICU culture
- Prioritization
- Lack of patient or family knowledge
- Patient or family refusal
- Safety concerns
- Patient fatigue
- Staffing
- Time constraints
- Lack of leadership
- Cost

*Data from* Refs.[5,11,21,23–26]

prevented.[8] Each patient scenario is unique and requires a personalized plan of care related to mobility, there is not a standard course of rehabilitation interventions appropriate for all. Critical thinking and problem-solving are needed skills to successfully overcome mobility barriers.

Sedation is another known barrier to ICU patient mobility. Sedative medications are commonly used in the ICU to enhance patient comfort but limiting their use has been directly shown to aid early mobilization success.[21] Higher doses of sedation decrease patient cognition and complicate their ability to actively participate in mobility exercises and appropriately follow commands.[22] Lighter sedation is recommended, even for patients with mechanical ventilation.[22] Lessening sedation allows for the patients to be more interactive with their environment and follow commands.[22] Increased ability to follow commands allows for more active participation in mobility activities. Nurses should frequently assess the need for sedation and use the smallest effective dose. With minimal sedation, activity participation in mobility interventions can increase and allow for better patient sleep.

## Overcoming Mobility Barriers

Barriers to early mobility interventions can and must be overcome.[19] Nurses are known to be problem solvers and they can collaborate with other members of the interdisciplinary team to plan and implement early mobilization and rehabilitation for their ICU patients (**Box 4**). Working together, the team can personalize plans of care and overcome specific patient mobility barriers while maintaining safety. Appropriate staffing, equipment, mobility prioritization, and education for staff, patients, and family members are essential to the long term success of ICU mobility.[26]

Lack of knowledge about the importance and benefits of early mobilization can be a barrier. Education of all patient care staff, the patient, and family about the need for mobility and established protocols can promote an ICU culture that supports early

---

**Box 4**
**Suggestions to overcome mobility barriers**

- Less sedative medications
- Passive movements when needed
- Staff education on mobility
- Detailed mobility protocols
- Patient education on mobility
- Family education on mobility
- Family engagement
- Adequate mobility equipment and training on it
- Dedicated physical therapist to the ICU
- Increased nurse staffing
- Strong leadership

*Data from* Schallom M, Tymkew H, Vyers K, Prentice D, Sona C, Norris T, Arroyo C. (2020). Implementation of an interdisciplinary AACN early mobility protocol. *Critical Care Nurse*, 2020;40(4):7-17 and Dubb R, Nydahl P, Hermes C, Schwabbauer N, Toonstra A, Parker AM, Kaltwasser A, Needham DM. Barriers and strategies for early mobilization of patients in intensive care units. *Annals of the American Thoracic Society.* 2016;13(5):724–730.

patient mobilization.[26] Hospitals can provide in-services and other educational opportunities for staff about the importance of mobility interventions to increase awareness, understanding, and implementation. ICU staff must prioritize early patient mobilization to prevent further complications during their hospital stay and promote sleep. ICU staff identifying the importance of early mobility is crucial in improving patient outcomes and quality of sleep.

Patient motivation, fatigue, and sleepiness are barriers that staff must accommodate. By including the patient or family members when possible, increased motivation and participation should result. Sleepiness can be improved with early mobility.[12] Encouraging patients to participate in mobility exercises can relieve feelings of daytime sleepiness.[12] Nurses can provide education on the link between mobility and sleep quality to increase patient motivation to actively participate in their mobility plan.

Higher sedation or acuity of patient illness may prevent active patient participation with mobility interventions. Nurses or other members of the health care team can assist with passive movements when active mobility interventions are not possible. PLEs that consist of moving a joint as tolerated is an early mobilization option for sedated or unconscious patients.[18]

A multidisciplinary approach to early and sustained mobility can increase success.[9] Multiple disciplines provide many different ways of viewing barriers and finding solutions for the ultimate outcome of improving patient mobility and sleep. Nurses frequently report mobility barriers as hemodynamic instability, whereas physical therapists report neurologic impairments and the inability to appropriately follow commands as what hinders early mobilization.[23] Collaboration within the interdisciplinary team is essential to successfully coordinating and completing patient rehabilitation programs.[9]

Physical therapy and early mobilization can be safely performed with critically ill patients.[9,20] Despite staff concerns, safety events are not common occurrences during mobility interventions.[8] Even though the benefits of early mobility and safety have been established, the overall number of ICU patients mobilized remains low.[9,27] Nurses and other members of the interdisciplinary care team can play a pivotal role in advocating and performing early mobility interventions with their ICU patients.

## SUMMARY

Patients in critical care face sleep challenges and a multitude of other potential complications. Early mobility is crucial to promoting sleep, minimizing risk for ICUAW, and preventing additional immobility based problems. Nurses and all ICU staff should advocate for mobility and push for its implementation daily. ICU mobility can be safely applied and personalized around specific patient challenges or barriers. An interdisciplinary approach to mobility programs, interventions, and goals allows for optimal patient outcomes. A culture that understands and fosters early mobility is needed to increase the number of ICU patients mobilized.

## CLINICS CARE POINTS

- Patient mobility in the ICU is safe
- Early mobility prevents numerous complications in critically ill patients
- Early mobility aids in falling asleep
- Increased mobility improves sleep quality
- ICU staff must prioritize, advocate, and implement patient mobility exercises

- Patient mobility in ICU needs to be increased
- Interdisciplinary approach to mobility in the ICU is recommended
- Barriers to mobility need to be evaluated to find safe strategies to its daily use

## DISCLOSURE

J. Rohr has nothing to disclose.

## REFERENCES

1. Zhang L, Hu W, Cai Z, et al. Early mobilization of critically ill patients in the intensive care unit: a systematic review and meta-analysis. PLoS One 2019;14(10): e0223185.
2. Ecklund MM, Bloss JW. Progressive mobility as a team effort in transitional care. Crit Care Nurse 2015;35(3):62–8.
3. Adler J, Malone D. Early mobilization in the intensive care unit: a systematic review. Cardiopulm Phys Ther J 2012;23(1):5–13.
4. Wu X, Li Z, Cao J, et al. The association between major complications of immobility during hospitalization and quality of life among bedridden patients: a 3 month prospective multi-center study. PLoS One 2018;13(10):e0205729.
5. Parry SM, Puthucheary ZA. The impact of extended bed rest on the musculoskeletal system in the critical care environment. Extrem Physiol Med 2015;4:16.
6. Hermans G, Van den Berghe G. Clinical review: intensive care unit acquired weakness. Crit Care 2015;19(1):274.
7. Morrison SA, Mirnik D, Korsic S, et al. Bed rest and hypoxic exposure affect sleep architecture and breathing stability. Front Physiol 2017;8:410.
8. Devlin JW, Skrobik Y, Gélinas C, et al. Clinical practice guidelines for the prevention and management of pain, agitation/sedation, delirium, immobility, and sleep disruption in adult patients in the ICU. Crit Care Med 2018;46(9):825–73.
9. Schallom M, Tymkew H, Vyers K, et al. (2020). Implementation of an interdisciplinary AACN early mobility protocol. Crit Care Nurse 2020;40(4):7–17.
10. Barnes-Daly MA, Pun BT, Harmon LA, et al. Improving health care for critically ill patients using an evidence-based collaborative approach to ABCDEF bundle dissemination and implementation. Worldviews Evid Based Nurs 2018;15(3): 206–16.
11. DeMellow JM, Kim TY, Romano PS, et al. Factors associated with ABCDE bundle adherence in critically ill adults requiring mechanical ventilation: an observational design. Intensive Crit Care Nurs 2020;60:102873.
12. Reade MC, Liu D. Optimising sleep in the ICU. ICU Manag Pract 2018;18(3): 200–4.
13. Dammeyer JA, Baldwin N, Packard D, et al. Mobilizing outcomes: implementation of a nurse-led multidisciplinary mobility program. Crit Care Nurs Q 2013;36(1): 109–19.
14. Sleep and sleep disorders, tips for better sleep. Centers for Disease Control and Prevention. July 15th, 2016. Available at: https://www.cdc.gov/sleep/about_ sleep/sleep_hygiene.html. Accessed October 30, 2020.
15. Tan X, Van Egmond L, Partinen M, et al. A narrative review of interventions for improving sleep and reducing circadian disruption in medical inpatients. Sleep Med 2019;59:42–50.

16. Jung AR, Park JI, Kim HS. Physical activity for prevention and management of sleep disturbances. Sleep Med Res 2020;11(1):15–8.

17. Alves A, Rabiais I, Nascimento M. Promoting interventions of sleep and comfort in intensive united care patients. Int J Nurs 2015;2(2):94–103.

18. Younis G, Sayed Ahmed S. Effectiveness of passive range of motion exercise on hemodynamic parameters and behavioral pain intensity among adult mechanically ventilated patients. IOSR Journal of Nursing and Health Science 2015; 4(6):47–59.

19. Denehy L, Lanphere J, Needham DM. Ten reasons why ICU patients should be mobilized early. Intensive Care Med 2017;43(1):86–90.

20. Fraser D, Spiva L, Forman W, et al. Original research: implementation of an early mobility program in an ICU. Am J Nurs 2015;115(12):49–58.

21. Shah FA, Girard TD, Yende S. Limiting sedation for patients with acute respiratory distress syndrome - time to wake up. Curr Opin Crit Care 2017;23(1):45–51.

22. Kress JP. Sedation and mobility: changing the paradigm. Crit Care Clin 2013; 29(1):67–75.

23. Hermes C, Nydahl P, Blobner M, et al. Assessment of mobilization capacity in 10 different ICU scenarios by different professions. PLoS One 2020;15(10): e0239853.

24. Pawlik A, Kress J. Issues affecting the delivery of physical therapy services for individuals with critical illness. Phys Ther 2013;93(2):256–65.

25. Hopkins RO, Spuhler VJ, Thomsen GE. Transforming ICU culture to facilitate early mobility. Crit Care Clin 2007;23(1):81–96.

26. Dubb R, Nydahl P, Hermes C, et al. Barriers and strategies for early mobilization of patients in intensive care units. Ann Am Thorac Soc 2016;13(5):724–30.

27. Engel HJ, Tatebe S, Alonzo PB, et al. Physical therapist–established intensive care unit early mobilization program: quality improvement project for critical care at the University of California San Francisco medical center. Phys Ther 2013;93(7):975–85.

# Effect of Opioids on Sleep

Karen Bergman Schieman, PhD, RN*,1, Jaime Rohr, MSN, RN-BC1

## KEYWORDS

- Opioids • Sleep • Intensive care unit • Withdrawal

## KEY POINTS

- Opioid medication is a first-line pain management in the intensive care unit for non-neuropathic pain.
- Opioids impact the quality of sleep.
- Opioids should be titrated to minimize withdrawal.

## INTRODUCTION

There are an estimated 25 million intensive care unit (ICU) days per year (Society of Critical Care Medicine). While in the ICU, analgesia and sedation are important treatments. Opioid analgesia is the first-line drug of choice for non-neuropathic pain in critically ill patients.[1] Herzig and colleagues[2] report that 51% of hospitalized patients in their study received opioid analgesics. Yaffe and associates[3] found that approximately 88% of patients hospitalized in the ICU settings were prescribed opioid medications.[3] Although their use is often necessary for the management of pain and comfort during procedures and care, there are side effects and consequences that must be addressed.

Nurses routinely assess pain levels and titrate medications for optimal effect. It is known that there are many side effects to opioid analgesia, including well-known ones such as respiratory depression and constipation; however, health care workers should be aware of lesser known side effects, such as sleep difficulties. Because of the numerous side effects, it is recommended that, when able, opioid medications be titrated down and nonopioid medications and alternative pain management techniques be used.

This article outlines the use of opioid analgesia in the ICU, and describes the short- and long-term effects of the medications on the patient's sleep quality. In addition, the need for monitoring and safety during the withdrawal of opioids are discussed. Last, considerations for discharging a patient from the ICU with regard to opioid use and sleep difficulties are addressed.

Bronson School of Nursing, Western Michigan University, Kalamazoo, MI, USA
1 Present address: 1903 W. Michigan Ave, Kalamazoo, MI 49008.
* Corresponding author.
E-mail address: karen.bergman@wmich.edu

Crit Care Nurs Clin N Am 33 (2021) 203–212
https://doi.org/10.1016/j.cnc.2021.01.003
0899-5885/21/© 2021 Elsevier Inc. All rights reserved.
ccnursing.theclinics.com

## REVIEW OF THE LITERATURE
### Opioid Impact on Sleep

Opioids can have both positive and negative impacts on sleep (**Table 1**). Pain that is poorly controlled interferes with sleep and can cause numerous complications in the ICU. The balance between pain control and side effects needs to be monitored closely. Sleep is vital to recovery and lack of sleep in the ICU has been linked to delirium, post-ICU syndrome, and increased length of stay in the hospital. In 2010, post-ICU syndrome was identified as a new condition that includes worsening of physical and cognitive status that arise after critical illness and last beyond the intensive care hospital stay.[4]

Conventional sleep cycles consist of both REM and non-REM. REM sleep makes up 20% to 25% of sleep and non-REM consists of 75% to 80%.[5] Robertson and associates[6] found that poor sleep quality was reported in 93% of individuals taking some form of opioid versus only 20% of the control group that did not take any form of opioids. Opioid sleep disturbances affect both REM and non-REM sleep. Studies have shown that opioid medications can decrease REM sleep by 50% and can also suppress deep non-REM sleep and increase light sleep.[7] Sleep disruptions can happen with opioid dependence, short- or long-term use, and even healthy individuals receiving acute administration can have altered sleep patterns.[7] This finding shows that, even with careful opioid administration by a health care professional, sleep disturbances can occur in the controlled ICU setting.

Although opioids are known to cause drowsiness, this effect does not lead to quality sleep patterns or feelings of restfulness. The negative impacts of opioids on sleep patterns include decreased total sleep time, increased sleep interruptions, and increased sleep onset latency.[8] Serdarevic and colleagues[9] found that opioid prescription use increases insomnia likelihood 42% compared with non-opioid use.

Mechanical ventilation is commonly needed and used in the ICU setting. Patients requiring mechanical ventilation receive opioids to foster comfort and ventilator use has been directly linked to sleep deprivation.[10] Based on this information, nurses can see that there is a relationship with the need for medications to tolerate mechanical ventilation and then the side effects of those medications negatively impacting sleep.

Nurses are in a unique position with the amount of time they spend with patients to help assess and limit sleep interruptions. Clustering nursing care activities together to allow periods of 90 to 120 minutes of uninterrupted sleep is recommended.[11] Nurses can not only cluster their care together, but limit unnecessary patient care interventions at night to help prevent interruptions in patient sleep patterns. Nurses are

**Table 1**
**Opioid sleep side effects**

| Negative | Positive |
|---|---|
| Daytime drowsiness | Restfulness |
| Sedation | Total sleep time |
| Non-REM sleep | Daytime alertness |
| Arousal during sleep attempts | REM sleep |
| Sleep latency | |
| Wakefulness after sleep onset | |
| Use of sleep aiding medications | |
| Patient reporting of sleep disturbances | |

Data from: Fathi H.R, Yoonessi A, Khatibi A, Rezaeitalab F, Rezaei-Ardani A. Crosstalk between sleep disturbance and opioid use disorder: A narrative review. Addiction & Health, 2020;12(2):140.

responsible for accurate assessment of patient comfort, management of pain, and also must consider the ramifications of nursing care and medication administration on sleep.

## Sleep Apnea

It is well-known that opioid use can cause respiratory depression, but a lesser known phenomenon is opioid drug's impact on sleep-disordered breathing (SDB). SDB encompasses both obstructive sleep apnea and central sleep apnea.[12] Obstructive sleep apnea is characterized by airways completely or partially closing during end-expiration while asleep.[13] Central sleep apnea is characterized by pauses in breathing during sleep from signal disruption by the central nervous system.[14] A range of breathing abnormalities besides apneas can occur with opioid use and include hypopnea, nocturnal hypoxia, ataxic breathing, and irregular breathing patterns.[15]

Opioid analgesics combined with benzodiazepines increase risk for SDB. The morphine-equivalent daily dose of opioids is associated with the development and severity of SDB and central sleep apnea.[16] Because of this, nurses should use their assessment skills along with standardized measurement tools for pain and sedation to provide comfort for the patient while mitigating the risk for SDB. A more detailed overview of sleep apnea in the ICU can be found in another section of this journal.

## Opioid Withdrawal and Sleep

Poor sleep can result from both opioid use and opioid withdrawal syndrome. Morphine use for 2 weeks results in withdrawal symptoms of greater sleep/wake transitions and increased NREM sleep.[7] The clinical significance of this withdrawal phenomenon is that, when critically ill patients are weaned from analgesics, their recovery can be slowed by increased amounts of sleepiness. When opioids are tapered or stopped, withdrawal symptoms can occur in mechanically ventilated critically ill patients with opioid use for longer than 72 hours. The higher the opioid dose and the longer length of use, the more the risk of withdrawal increases.[17]

Opioid withdrawal can be broken down into 2 phases, the initial or acute phase, and the chronic phase.[18] In the hospitalized patient, it is more common to see patients exhibiting signs of the acute phase, including agitation, anxiety, dysphoria, insomnia, and temperature instability.[18] More than 50% of patients will experience withdrawal symptoms after 5 days of opioid use, and 100% after 9 days if opioids are withdrawn.[19]

In the hospital setting when opioids are withdrawn nurses need to assess for iatrogenic withdrawal syndrome (IWS). IWS can result from discontinuing or weaning opioids and is characterized by overstimulation of the central nervous system, autonomic dysregulation, and gastrointestinal symptoms. Symptoms of IWS are shown in **Box 1**, and can include mental, physical, and emotional disturbances. Patients experiencing IWS and increased wakefulness while in the ICU setting have additional sleep challenges. The gastrointestinal symptoms that accompany opioid withdrawal can also make sleep difficult. Nausea, vomiting, cramping, and diarrhea are common and can pose many challenges to falling asleep or staying asleep if left untreated. The management of IWS symptoms is essential to promote healthier sleep patterns.

IWS can develop in patient populations of all ages. Adult intensive care patients have an IWS incidence rate of 32% and in pediatric intensive care patients, it can be up to 57%.[17] IWS needs to be identified early but this can pose a significant clinical challenge owing to the potential overlaps in conditions. Larosa and associates[19] found that infections, metabolic derangements, cerebrovascular insults, encephalopathy, hypoxia, hypercarbia, delirium, psychosis, and inadequate sedation are all conditions

---

**Box 1**
**IWS symptoms**

Central nervous system stimulation
  Agitation
  Irritability
  Tremors
  Increased wakefulness

Sympathetic nervous system hyperactivation
  Hypertension
  Tachycardia
  Fever
  Sweating

Gastrointestinal disturbances
  Nausea
  Vomiting
  Loose stools
  Diarrhea

*Data from*: Wang PP, Huang E, Feng X, Bray CA, Perreault MM, Rico P, Bellemare P, Murgoi P, Gélinas C, Lecavalier A, Jayaraman D. Opioid-associated iatrogenic withdrawal in critically ill adult patients: A multicenter prospective observational study. *Annals of Intensive Care*, 2017;7(1):1-7.

---

that need to be considered and ruled out when IWS is suspected. Once IWS is identified accurately, treatment can begin. Gradual opioid weaning, recognizing and treating withdrawal-specific symptoms, and the administration of needed rescue therapies are recommended IWS treatment.[19] Methadone is commonly used as a first-line choice for IWS owing to its mechanism of action and favorable pharmacokinetics.[19] Methadone is long acting and can help to manage IWS symptoms without the patient experiencing the highs and lows associated with shorter acting opioids.[20]

Physical examination can provide cues to opioid withdrawal. Symptoms of withdrawal can be objective or subjective. Objective findings that can be identified with physical assessments include mydriasis, tachycardia, hypertension, diaphoresis, and piloerection.[21] Subjective findings can include patient or family reporting of symptoms. Nursing considerations for IWS include close monitoring, identifying high-risk patients, obtaining a drug use history, and assessing signs and symptoms. Some of the risks for IWS are intuitive, such as high-dose opioids and longer duration of use. Others are lesser known, such as high body mass index, respiratory distress syndrome, septic shock, and young age. Familiarizing oneself with the risk factors for IWS can help nurses identify the condition early and accurately and initiate treatment promptly.

### Opioid Withdrawal Assessment

A tool used to assess opioid withdrawal severity is the Clinical Opioid Withdrawal Scale (COWS), which consists of 11 items with different scoring based on symptom severity.[22] Numerous symptoms are outlined in detail on the COWS scale that are thought to pose complications to restful sleep. **Table 2** provides a detailed description of the symptoms assessed by the COWS scale.

After the COWS scale is completed and the score compiled, the numerical value is used to indicate opioid withdrawal symptom severity. COWS classifies withdrawals as mild, moderate, moderately severe, or severe (**Table 3**).[22]

**Table 2**
Symptoms assessed by the COWS scale

| COWS Question | 0 | 1 | 2 | 3 | 4 | 5 |
|---|---|---|---|---|---|---|
| Resting pulse rate beats/minute | Pulse rate 80 or below | Pulse rate 81–100 | Pulse Rate 101–120 | X | Pulse rate >120 | X |
| Sweating | No reports of chills or flushing | Subjective report of chills or flushing | Flushed or observable moistness on face | Beads of sweat on brow or face | Sweat streaming off face | X |
| Restlessness | Able to sit still | Reports difficulty sitting still, but able to | X | Frequent shifting or extraneous movements of arms/legs | X | Unable to sit still for more than a few seconds |
| Pupil size | Pinned or normal for size for room light | Possibly larger than normal for room light | Moderately dilated | X | X | So dilated that only the rim is visible |
| Bone or joint aches | Not present | Mild diffuse discomfort | Patient reports severe diffuse aching of joint/muscles | X | Patient is rubbing joints or muscles and is unable to sit still from discomfort | X |
| Runny nose or tearing | Not present | Nasal stuffiness or unusually moist eyes | Nose running or tearing | X | Nose constantly running or tears down cheeks | X |
| GI upset | No GI symptoms | Stomach cramps | Nausea or loose stools | Vomiting or diarrhea | X | Multiple episodes of diarrhea or vomiting |
| Tremor | No tremor | Tremor is felt but not observed | Slight tremor observable | X | Gross tremor or muscle twitching | X |

(continued on next page)

**Table 2**
*(continued)*

| COWS Question | 0 | 1 | 2 | 3 | 4 | 5 |
|---|---|---|---|---|---|---|
| Yawning | No yawning | Yawning once or twice during assessment | Yawning 3 or more times during assessment | X | Yawning several times per minute | X |
| Anxiety or irritability | None | Patient reports increasing anxiousness or irritability | Obviously irritable or anxious | X | So irritable or anxious that participation is assessment is difficult | X |
| Gooseflesh Skin | Smooth skin | X | X | Piloerection of skin felt or hairs standing up on arms | X | Prominent piloerection |

*Abbreviation:* GI, gastrointestinal.

Donald R. Wesson & Walter Ling (2003) The Clinical Opiate Withdrawal Scale (COWS), Journal of Psychoactive Drugs, 35:2, 253-259, https://doi.org/10.1080/02791072.2003.10400007; with permission.

| Table 3 Opioid withdrawal symptom severity | |
|---|---|
| Cows Score | Symptom Severity |
| 0–4 | No significant withdrawal |
| 5–12 | Mild withdrawal |
| 13–24 | Moderate withdrawal |
| 25–36 | Moderately severe withdrawal |
| >36 | Severe withdrawal |

*Data from* Canamo & Tronco. Clinical Opioid Withdrawal Scale (COWS): Implementation and outcomes. *Critical Care Nursing Quarterly,* 2019;42(3):222-226.

Two other opioid withdrawal scales can be used in the inpatient setting in addition to the COWS. The subjective opioid withdrawal scale (SOWS) is a 16 item subjective assessment tool, and the short opioid withdrawal scale-Gossop (SOWS-Gossop) are both available to assess the severity of opioid withdrawal.[18] The assessment tool used depends on organizational policy.

### Weaning Opioids

Monitored the weaning of opioids can decrease the symptoms associated with IWS and minimize sleep-related problems. As mentioned elsewhere in this article, withdrawal can occur with the use of opioids for more than 5 days. The weaning of opioids should take place when dependence is known or suspected (**Box 2**). The goal when removing opioid therapy is to minimize withdrawal symptoms while finding a way to prevent pain flare ups in patients who suffer from chronic pain.[23]

Opioids are commonly used in critically ill patients, but the amount and frequency needed should decrease as the patient stabilizes. Hospitalized patients who were receiving decreased opioid doses started to experience opioid withdrawal symptoms 24 hours after their dose was less than 50% of the maximal dose.[24] Arroyo-Novoa and

---

**Box 2**
**Nursing considerations for when to wean opioids**

- Patient request
- No pain reduction
- No function improvement
- Adverse effects that are unmanageable
- Unsafe behaviors (early refills, lost pills, buying/borrowing opioids)
- Concerns for substance use disorder
- Opioid overdose
- High-risk comorbidities (chronic obstructive pulmonary disease, sleep apnea, liver disease, addiction history, advanced age, fall risk)
- Concurrent use with benzodiazepines
- Worsening mental health comorbidities (post-traumatic stress disorder, anxiety, depression)

*Data from*: Opioid taper decision tool. U.S. Department of Veterans Affairs. *A VA Clinician's Guide.* October 2016, accessed September 25th, 2020. https://www.pbm.va.gov/AcademicDetailingService/Documents/Pain_Opioid_Taper_Tool_IB_10_939_P96820.pdf.

associates[25] recommend weaning the dose of opioid infusion in the ICU by 10% per day. This recommendation is not appropriate for everyone and personalization of the treatment plan may be needed. Patients with a history of drug use disorders may require different tapering regimens.[25]

### Considerations for Discharge

Prolonged time in the ICU has been linked to potential problems including sleep disturbances (Tiruvoipati).[26] Pain control is a priority in the ICU, but that does not mean opioids are the only answer. Adjunctive medications for sedation and pain control should be used in the ICU to limit opioid use. Zhao and associates[27] found that acetaminophen, ketamine, nonsteroidal anti-inflammatory drugs, and neuropathic pain medications can all help to decrease opioid overuse.

Patients who have uncontrolled pain at discharge may need to leave the hospital with an opioid prescription. Stamenkovic and colleagues[28] found that 12.2% of patients at discharge were still using opioids. Owing to the highly addictive nature of opioids, patient education and follow-up are key. Opioid use should be discontinued when possible and with the supervision of a health care professional.

The opioid epidemic has raised awareness regarding the overprescribing of controlled substances and highlighted the need for close monitoring for patients discharged home with opioid analgesics. In 2012, the national averages for opioid prescriptions dispensed was in excess of 255 million, at a rate of 81.3 prescriptions for every 100 persons.[29] The latest reported numbers are from 2018 and the opioid prescriptions have declined to a national average of 51.4 for every 100 persons.[29] This prescribing rate equates to about 168 million opioid prescriptions in total.[29]

In an ideal world, opioids would be weaned while in the hospital and this would decrease dependence on these medications. In the real world, people will require opioids at discharge, but a conversation between the patient and the health care providers should stress the importance of continuing the weaning process while implementing alternative therapies for pain management. Patients leaving the hospital with a prescription for opioids should know the potential for addiction as well as the side effects of the medications, including sleep disturbance.

### SUMMARY

Opioid medications are often necessary for the comfort of patients in the ICU. Although patients may seem to be sleeping, the quality of their sleep may be impacted by the medications they are receiving. Nurses and health care workers can carefully assess and manage patients so that opioid medications are used judiciously for comfort while limiting their overuse or long-term use. When withdrawing opioids from the patient in the ICU, monitoring with tools such as the COWS scale is recommended and abrupt removal of opioid medication after long term use is to be avoided. If patients require opioid medications at discharge, thoughtful discussions should occur between health care providers and patients about the side effects, including sleep disturbance, and the risk for addiction.

### CLINICS CARE POINTS

- Opioid medications cause drowsiness; however, the quality of sleep is impaired.
- Nurses should assess for SDB in patients receiving opioid medications.
- Opioids use should be monitored, and weaning should occur when possible.
- IWS can occur when opioids are withdrawn too quickly.

## DISCLOSURE

K.B. Schieman and J. Rohr have nothing to disclose.

## REFERENCES

1. Barr J, Fraser GL, Puntillo K, et al. Clinical practice guidelines for the management of pain, agitation, and delirium in adult patients in the intensive care unit. Am Coll Crit Care Med 2013;41(1):263–306.
2. Herzig SJ, Rothberg MB, Cheung M, et al. Opioid utilization and opioid-related adverse events in nonsurgical patients in US hospitals. J Hosp Med 2014;9(2): 73–81.
3. Yaffe PB, Green RS, Butler MB, et al. Is admission to the intensive care unit associated with chronic opioid use? A 4-year follow-up of intensive care unit survivors. J Intensive Care Med 2017;32(7):429–35.
4. Fuke R, Hifumi T, Kondo Y, et al. Early rehabilitation to prevent postintensive care syndrome in patients with critical illness: a systematic review and meta-analysis. BMJ Open 2018;8(5):e019998.
5. Rittayamai N, Wilcox E, Drouot X, et al. Positive and negative effects of mechanical ventilation on sleep in the ICU: a review with clinical recommendations. Intensive Care Med 2016;42(4):531–41.
6. Robertson J, Purple R, Cole P, et al. Sleep disturbance in patients taking opioid medication for chronic back pain. Anaesthesia 2016;71(11):1296–307.
7. Eacret D, Veasey SC, Blendy JA. Bidirectional relationship between opioids and disrupted sleep: putative mechanisms. Mol Pharmacol 2020;98(2):445–53.
8. Angarita GA, Emadi N, Hodges S, et al. Sleep abnormalities associated with alcohol, cannabis, cocaine, and opioid use: a comprehensive review. Addict Sci Clin Pract 2016;11(1):1–17.
9. Serdarevic M, Osborne V, Striley CW, et al. The association between insomnia and prescription opioid use: results from a community sample in Northeast Florida. Sleep Health 2017;3(5):368–72.
10. White B, Zomorodi M. Perceived and actual noise levels in critical care units. Intensive Crit Care Nurs 2017;38:18–23.
11. Uğraş GA, Babayigit S, Tosun K, et al. The effect of nocturnal patient care interventions on patient sleep and satisfaction with nursing care in neurosurgery intensive care unit. J Neurosci Nurs 2015;47(2):104–12.
12. Khayat R, Abraham W. Current treatment approaches and trials in central sleep apnea. Int J Cardiol 2016;206(SS):22–7.
13. Hashemian SMR, Kassiri N. Sleep disorders in critical care unit. J Pulmonol Clin Res 2018;1:1–4.
14. American Sleep Association. Sleep apnea; 2020. Available at: https://www.sleepassociation.org/sleep-apnea/. Accessed October 1, 2020.
15. Davis M, Mehta Z. Opioids and chronic pain: where is the balance? Curr Oncol Rep 2016;18(12):1–14.
16. Correa D, Farney RJ, Chung F, et al. Chronic opioid use and central sleep apnea: a review of the prevalence, mechanisms, and perioperative considerations. Anesth Analg 2015;120(6):1273–85.
17. Wang PP, Huang E, Feng X, et al. Opioid-associated iatrogenic withdrawal in critically ill adult patients: a multicenter prospective observational study. Ann Intensive Care 2017;7(1):1–7.
18. Prunty LM, Prunty JJ. Acute opioid withdrawal: identification and treatment strategies. US Pharmacist 2016;41(11):2–6.

19. LaRosa JM, Aponte-Patel L. Iatrogenic withdrawal syndrome: a review of patho-physiology, prevention, and treatment. Curr Pediatr Rep 2019;7(1):12–9.
20. Woods JS, Joseph H. From narcotic to normalizer: the misperception of metha-done treatment and the persistence of prejudice and bias. Subst Use Misuse 2018;53(2):323–9.
21. Duber HC, Barata IA, Cioè-Peña E, et al. Identification, management, and transi-tion of care for patients with opioid use disorder in the emergency department. Ann Emerg Med 2018;72(4):420–31.
22. Canamo L, Tronco N. Clinical Opioid Withdrawal Scale (COWS): implementation and outcomes. Crit Care Nurs Q 2019;42(3):222–6.
23. Agarwal V, Louw A, Puentedura E. Physician-delivered pain neuroscience educa-tion for opioid tapering: a case report. Int J Environ Res Public Health 2020;17(9): 3324.
24. Hyun D, Huh J, Hong S, et al. Iatrogenic opioid withdrawal syndrome in critically ill patients: a retrospective cohort study. J Korean Med Sci 2020;35(15):106.
25. Arroyo-Novoa CM, Figueroa-Ramos MI, Puntillo KA. Opioid and benzodiazepine iatrogenic withdrawal syndrome in patients in the intensive care unit. AACN Adv Crit Care 2019;30(4):353–64.
26. Tiruvoipati R, Botha J, Fletcher J, et al. Intensive care discharge delay is associ-ated with increased hospital length of stay: A multicentre prospective observa-tional study. PloS One 2017;12(7):E0181827.
27. Zhao H, Yang S, Wang H, et al. Non-opioid analgesics as adjuvants to opioid for pain management in adult patients in the ICU: a systematic review and meta-analysis. J Crit Care 2019;54:136–44.
28. Stamenkovic DM, Laycock H, Karanikolas M, et al. Chronic pain and chronic opioid use after intensive care discharge - is it time to change practice? Front Pharmacol 2019;10:23.
29. U.S. Opioid prescribing rate Maps. Centers for disease control and prevention. 2020. Available at: https://www.cdc.gov/drugoverdose/maps/rxrate-maps.html. Accessed October 1st, 2020.

# To Sleep, or Not to Sleep, that Is the Question

Glenn Carlson, MSN, ACNP-BC[a],[1],*, Alyssa Curtis, RN, BSN[b],[1]

## KEYWORDS

- Sleep • Guideline • Protocol • ICU • Sleep disruption

## KEY POINTS

- Sleep disruptions occur in the intensive care unit and affect outcomes of length of stay, delirium days, and long-term cognition.
- Implementation of a sleep hygiene protocol should use structured quality improvement and implementation plans.
- There are many risk factors for the development of sleep disruption.
- Pharmacologic and nonpharmacologic interventions to prevent sleep disruption are available.

## INTRODUCTION

Construction of a sleep hygiene guideline/protocol is complex because of the difficulty in measuring quality of sleep or sleep disruptions as observed, or the more expensive and resource-intensive objective measurement via polysomnography.[1–4] In addition, the literature regarding what causes disruption, what places patient at risk for disruption, and interventions designed to limit disruption and promote sleep has inconsistent results.[1–8] Last, the effect of sleep on a variety of outcomes, such as delirium, intensive care unit (ICU) length of stay (LOS), hospital LOS, and mortality, is also inconclusive in many cases. Development of a sleep hygiene guideline uses the best possible evidence while reevaluating frequently as new evidence become available. Employing a successful sleep hygiene guideline should use a structured quality improvement model and structured implementation plan.

## APPROACH

Utilization of a structured assessment and implementation program is the best way to ensure implementation and sustainability of a sleep protocol over time. Use of the

a Division of Critical Care and Pulmonary Medicine, Bronson Battle Creek, Battle Creek, MI 49107, USA; b Bronson Battle Creek, Battle Creek, MI 49107, USA
1 Present address: 300 North Avenue. Battle Creek, MI 48197.
* Corresponding author.
*E-mail address:* carlsong@bronsonhg.org
Twitter: @GlennICU (G.C.); @alyssacurtis33 (A.C.)

Crit Care Nurs Clin N Am 33 (2021) 213–217
https://doi.org/10.1016/j.cnc.2021.01.004
0899-5885/21/© 2021 Elsevier Inc. All rights reserved.

ccnursing.theclinics.com

OPDCA: Observe, Plan, Do, Check, Act model is an excellent quality improvement initiative that can accomplish success.

### Observe

Observe current conditions while seeking out and engaging team members for planning. Team members that are essential include the following:

1. Management and other leadership support
2. Peer bedside RN staff
3. Physician/provider support
4. Psychiatry, if available
5. Pharmacy representative
6. Respiratory therapy support

Cause of sleep disruption can be ascertained by questioning staff, patients, and families. Use the results of these surveys and compare the best available evidence for synergy. These observations form the basis for the beginning of implementing a plan for change.

### Plan/Do

See an opportunity based on your observations and formulate a plan. The plan should also be structured. The *Use of the Influencer, The Power to Change Anything*[4] has been used by several organizations to employ change successfully. The *Influencer* uses 6 sources of influence to enact change. Each source should be part of the implementation plan. The more sources that are used, the more successful the implementation. The 6 sources are as follows:

*Source 1: Personal Motivation*, whether you want to do it. Set up motivation for others to want to implement change.
*Source 2: Personal Ability*, whether you can do it. Ensure that the interventions are educated on and that they can easily be performed.
*Source 3: Social Motivation*, whether other people encourage the right behaviors. Use peer to peer support. Have peers do measurement and data collection.
*Source 4: Social Ability*, whether other people provide help, information, or resources. Involve as many health care provider groups as possible in the planning and intervention so there is more institutional buy-in.
*Source 5: Structural Motivation*, whether the environment encourages the right behaviors. Structure the environment to make the intervention as easy as possible. It is easy enough that people must do something outside their routines to avoid the intervention. Create posters with the interventions, add interventions to the electronic medical record (EMR), and make laminated cards with the interventions and hand them out to all health care team members.
*Source 6: Structural Ability*, whether the environment supports the right behaviors. This is where management and other leadership are helpful to ensure resources are available to support these interventions. Also, provide awards for successful and accountability milestones.

Interventions should be based on resolving issues or risk for sleep disruption. ICU patients have known risk factors for sleep disruptions, such as noise, light, nighttime interventions, vital sign measurement, anxiety/fear, and pain/discomfort[1-7] (**Box 1** lists these and other risk factors). Therefore, planning interventions to limit disruption should at minimum include these known risk factors. **Box 2** lists both nonpharmacologic and pharmacologic interventions to minimize disruptions.

---

**Box 1**
**Risks for sleep disruption**

Physiologic
1. Pain/discomfort
2. Coughing, breathing difficulty, hypoxemia/alkalosis
3. Thirst/hunger
4. Home sleep disturbance due to obstructive sleep apnea

Environmental
1. Restricted movement or immobility
2. Comfort of bed
3. Nursing interventions
4. Nocturnal pressure support ventilation
5. Light/sound
6. Nursing interventions

Iatrogenic
1. Medications, such as benzodiazepine and propofol
2. Ventilator asynchrony
3. Daytime sleep (one-half of ICU patients sleep occurs during the daytime3,6)

Psychological
1. Anxiety
2. Fear
3. Delirium

*Data from* Refs.[1–7]

---

An additional part of the plan is to select outcomes to measure that are feasible and are reliable and valid tools. The outcome to select should be a way to measure success of interventions enacted. Examples of outcomes to measure are delirium-free days, patient's perception of sleep, daytime sleepiness (Epworth Sleepiness Scale[1]), ICU LOS, medical device–free days, or less sedative use. Two additional reliable and valid tools for outcome measurement of sleep are the following:

1. Richard Campbell's Sleep Questionnaire[6,7]
2. Sleep ICU Questionnaire

---

**Box 2**
**Pharmacologic and nonpharmacologic interventions**

Nonpharmacologic intervention to prevent sleep disruption/fragmentation
1. Up during day, lights on, family visitation
2. Low light at night
3. Provision of an uninterrupted sleep time limiting interventions by staff
4. Assist control ventilation at night instead of pressure support[6]
5. Use of non invasive ventilation (NIV) when needed for obstructive sleep apnea
6. Limit use of restraint
7. Positioning of patient as would sleep at home
8. Ear plugs if patient prefers silence at night
9. Use of eye mask if patient prefers darkness

Pharmacologic intervention to promote sleep and prevent disruption/fragmentation
1. Melatonin[9,10]
2. Ramelteon[9]
3. Suvorexant[9]
4. Dexmedetomidine[9]
5. Minimize propofol/benzodiazepines[1,2]

Other outcomes to measure may include what effect sleep disruptions can have on delirium, ICU LOS, and mortality. Because delirium affects ICU and hospital LOS, mortality, post-ICU post traumatic stress disorder development, and post-ICU syndrome, many studies have used delirium as a surrogate for promotion of sleep. Promoting sleep decreases incidence of delirium and sleep is less when patients have delirium. Interestingly, many of the risk factors associated with sleep disruption and the interventions to promote sleep are synonymous with risk and prevention of delirium.[6]

Finally, set up measures of successful implementation, like observances and documentation of noise levels throughout the day, light levels throughout the day, use of earplugs/eye masks as needed, documentation of pain levels, or restraint use. Have an observable way to measure each intervention.

### Check

Check the data. Have interventions been completely enacted? Are measurements of outcome showing improvement? One way is to integrate the sleep hygiene guideline into the EMR. Reports can then be created from your EMR.

### Act

Take action on whatever did not work or an intervention that was not completely enacted. Also, take action on what did work in order to further improvement in those areas.

### IMPLICATIONS FOR FUTURE NURSING RESEARCH AND CLINICAL PRACTICE

Bedside nurses are positioned to affect many outcomes for ICU patients. Assessment of sleep patterns and disruptions has been studied, but results are inconsistent. The bedside nurse's observation of sleep in the ICU and disruptions for sleep needs more comprehensive and consistent research in order to optimize sleep. Also, an assessment of how sleep disruption affects long-term outcomes from ICU stay to after discharge home is needed. An adage that has been used that "sleep happens after discharge and not in the ICU" probably has a detrimental effect on long-term outcomes. Therefore, sleep hygiene in the ICU may be in its infancy, but its affect will be long lasting.

### SUMMARY

Polysomnography has shown that ICU sleep is quite fragmented or disrupted even though total sleep time was similar to non-ICU patients.[3,6] There are many risk factors for disrupted sleep and interventions to mitigate these risks. Using a structured quality improvement program can ensure success and sustainability of an ICU sleep hygiene guideline. Using an ICU sleep hygiene guideline can have a profound effect on patients both in the ICU and when discharged home. One study showed use of an ICU diary improved sleep at home after discharge.[11] The use of an ICU diary may also be an intervention to use as a part of a transition-to-home plan. The goal of the ICU sleep hygiene guideline should mirror all the provided care in the ICU in that critical care is not just in saving a life but also is promoting a lifetime. Using pharmacologic and nonpharmacologic interventions in a sleep guideline improves care in the ICU and optimizes functional ability when home.

### CLINICS CARE POINTS

- Sleep disruptions affect many outcomes in the hospital and long term.

- A structured quality improvement plan will ensure success and sustainability.
- Protocols should include interventions that minimize or eliminate sleep disruption.

## DISCLOSURE

G. Carlson and A. Curtis have nothing to disclose.

## REFERENCES

1. Honarmand K, Rafay H, Le J, et al. A systematic review of risk factors for sleep disruption in critically ill adults. Crit Care Med 2020. https://doi.org/10.1097/ccm.0000000000004405.
2. Devlin JW, Skrobik Y, Gélinas C, et al. Clinical practice guidelines for the prevention and management of pain, agitation/sedation, delirium, immobility, and sleep disruption in adult patients in the ICU. Crit Care Med 2018;46(9). https://doi.org/10.1097/ccm.0000000000003299.
3. Telias I, Wilcox ME. Sleep and circadian rhythm in critical illness. Crit Care 2019; 23(1). https://doi.org/10.1186/s13054-019-2366-0.
4. Patterson K, Grenny J, Maxfield D, et al. Use of influence, the power to change anything. New York: McGraw-Hill; 2007.
5. Elías MN, Munro CL, Liang Z, et al. Nighttime sleep duration is associated with length of stay outcomes among older adult survivors of critical illness. Dimensions Crit Care Nurs 2020;39(3):145–54.
6. Pisani MA, D'Ambrosio C. Sleep and delirium in adults who are critically ill. Chest 2020;157(4):977–84.
7. Romagnoli S, Villa G, Fontanarosa L, et al. Sleep duration and architecture in non-intubated intensive care unit patients: an observational study. Sleep Med 2020; 70:79–87.
8. Flannery AH, Oyler DR, Weinhouse GL. The impact of interventions to improve sleep on delirium in the ICU. Crit Care Med 2016;44(12):2231–40.
9. Fontaine GV, Nigoghossian CD, Hamilton LA. Melatonin, ramelteon, suvorexant, and dexmedetomidine to promote sleep and prevent delirium in critically ill patients: a narrative review with practical applications. Crit Care Nurs Q 2020; 43(2):232–50.
10. Lewandowska K, Małkiewicz MA, Siemiński M, et al. The role of melatonin and melatonin receptor agonist in the prevention of sleep disturbances and delirium in intensive care unit – a clinical review. Sleep Med 2020;69:127–34.
11. Wang S, Xin H, Vico CC, et al. Effect of an ICU diary on psychiatric disorders, quality of life, and sleep quality among adult cardiac surgical ICU survivors: a randomized controlled trial. Crit Care 2020;24(1). https://doi.org/10.1186/s13054-020-2797-7.

# Family Presence and Sleep in the Intensive Care Unit

Karen Bergman Schieman, PhD, RN

## KEYWORDS

- Family presence • Sleep • ICU

## KEY POINTS

- Patients report that they want their family at the bedside.
- Families fill multiple roles while at the bedside.
- Nurses can promote patient and family sleep.

## INTRODUCTION

Sleep is important to all people and is of special concern when it comes to hospitalized patients. The hospital environment is often not conducive to a restful night's sleep, and given that patients may stay for several days, the lack of sleep can accumulate to cause numerous detrimental effects.[1] Patients in the intensive care unit (ICU) environment may have even more difficulty with sleep due to the nature of care being given around the clock, increased noise from monitors, and discomfort from machines such as ventilators.[1]

The Society of Critical Care Medicine published "Clinical Practice Guidelines for the Prevention and Management of Pain, Agitation/Sedation, Delirium, Immobility, and Sleep Disruption in Adult Patients in the ICU" where they describe the common sleep disturbances of the ICU patient.[2] Sleep difficulties are characterized by fragmented sleep, more time spent in light sleep stages, and more time spent sleeping during daytime hours. Although total sleep time may be normal, the abnormal rapid eye movement and nonrapid eye movement sleep patterns are not conducive to restorative sleep. Together these sleep difficulties disrupt normal circadian rhythms and can affect healing, morbidity, and mortality.[2]

Sleep is important to restore energy needed for recovery of the hospitalized patient. Lack of restorative sleep can lead to cognitive dysfunction and delirium, which can result in worse outcomes.[3] Insufficient sleep can also cause problems with immune function, thermoregulation, metabolism, and pulmonary function.[3] Patients in the ICU cannot afford to experience these disruptions in their body functions while they are trying to survive critical illness.

Western Michigan University, 1903 W. Michigan Ave, Kalamazoo Mi, 49008, USA
*E-mail address:* Karen.bergman@wmich.edu

Crit Care Nurs Clin N Am 33 (2021) 219–224
https://doi.org/10.1016/j.cnc.2021.04.002
0899-5885/21/© 2021 Elsevier Inc. All rights reserved.

ccnursing.theclinics.com

Sleep in the ICU environment can be difficult, and the causes are 2-fold with environmental and person factors. The environment in the ICU tends to be noisy with monitors and alarms, bright lights for health care workers to perform their duties, and small rooms with multiple pieces of equipment and people. Person factors include anxiety, fear, pain, and unpredictable patient care interruptions.[4]

The purpose of this paper is to describe the effects of having a family member at the bedside of an ICU patient and the impact that it has on both the patient's and the family member's ability to sleep. The implication of a family member at the bedside on nursing care will also be addressed.

## IS A FAMILY MEMBER AT THE BEDSIDE BENEFICIAL TO THE PATIENT?

Positive results of families at the bedside of an ICU patient are summarized in a chapter of the book "Families in the Intensive Care Unit" by G. Netzer.[5] Some of the highlighted benefits include assisting with early mobilization, which is known to reduce length of stay, and having family at the bedside can reduce anxiety and ICU delirium. Families know the patient well and can help to detect when there are changes in status based on their knowledge of the patient's baseline status.[5]

Patients report visits from families/family presence as highly important in their ICU stay.[6] Family members are able to perform multiple roles including active presence, patient protector, facilitator, historian, coach, and voluntary caregiver.[7] According to McAdam's qualitative findings about family contributions in the ICU, these family roles are often underrecognized and underappreciated by ICU staff. Families are able to perform activities of daily living, which may relieve the ICU staff of some of those duties and free their time for more critical tasks. Families reported wanting to be physically close to their loved ones, and providing care such as massaging, repositioning, and communicating with the patient can help the family feel a sense of success while also assisting with the care responsibilities.[7]

## IMPLICATION OF STAYING OVERNIGHT IN THE INTENSIVE CARE UNIT ON THE FAMILY

Families have a strong desire to stay with their loved ones while in the ICU in order to provide comfort and support. Given that families want to stay and patients report it as beneficial, it seems logical that a family member would want to spend the night with the patient. A family member staying overnight is not without risks to the family member in terms of sleep deprivation. Families will be subjected to the same lights and noise that the patient is, and this can limit their ability to obtain a restful night's sleep.[5]

Families play an important role in care and support for their loved ones while the patient is in the ICU. Family, for the purpose of this article, will denote anyone who is supportive and is a significant person in the life of the patient. Roles of family members of hospitalized patients have been described as protector, coach, facilitator, historian, and volunteer caregiver.[7]

Netzer and colleagues[5] describe a phenomenon called family intensive care unit syndrome, including the 6 components of maladaptive reasoning, personal and family conflicts, cognitive bias, high-intensity emotions, anticipatory grief, and sleep deprivation. Verceles[8] report that half of family members of ICU patients report excessive daytime sleepiness. At the same time that they are sleep deprived, families are asked to absorb new information about the patient's status and make important decisions. One can see how the lack of sleep could further increase the stress of families trying to be supportive on an ongoing basis.

Families seek comfort themselves when in the ICU, and those needs may not be met.[9] Adequate sleep contributes to overall comfort. Owen's article about a Model of Family-Centered Care makes an important observation that families are exposed to the same lights and sounds in the ICU as the patient, but the patient likely gets sedation, ear plugs, and maybe eye masks.[10] With education, families can become knowledgeable about the importance of sleep for both the patient and themselves and can play an active role in promoting sleep for normal circadian rhythms. Families can help monitor the light in the room, ensuring lights are on during daytime and dim at night, mobility is promoted, and a quiet environment at night. Owen suggests that families be educated about their own sleep hygiene and recommend including information about the sleep environment, napping, and comfort measures for sleep. Families could be offered ear plugs and eye masks and a specific location for them to create a comfortable sleep environment.[10]

In the book "Families in the Intensive Care Unit," authors Jaiswal and Owens describe family's difficulty sleeping as 2-fold: (1) the lack of opportunity to sleep or (2) insomnia.[11] Lack of opportunity can have much to do with the ICU environment of small spaces, noises, lights, alarms, and so on. Families are often sleeping in chairs or small pull-out beds, which may not be comfortable enough for a restful night's sleep. Insomnia is the inability to fall asleep, stay asleep, or nonrestorative sleep often caused by stress, anxiety, or heightened emotions of the ICU family. In addition, financial burdens can weight on families while they are often out of town, away from work and other family members, eating meals at the hospital, all of which increase the stress they experience.[11]

Few studies have measured the amount of sleep obtained by family members of hospitalized patients. Choi and colleagues[12] studied 28 family caregivers' sleep quality when a loved one was admitted to the ICU and found that the Pittsburg Sleep Quality Index (PSQI) scores were elevated both while the patient was in the ICU as well as up to 2 months postdischarge. PSQI scores range from 0 to 21 with scores greater than 5 indicating poor sleep quality, and the higher the scores the worse the sleep quality. Caregivers reported PSQI with a mean of 6.9 while their family member was in the ICU, which decreased to 6.2 at 2 months postdischarge. They also report being awake at least an hour during the night and that they average about 5.5 hours of sleep while the patient is in the ICU.[12]

Celic and colleagues found an association with anxiety, depression, and fatigue of family members of ICU patients. In their study, 85% of families said "no" to the question about if their own care needs were attended to. They report that 348 out of 350 family members reported sleep problems, with 76% having moderate to severe problems. Their sample also reported high levels of anxiety (81%) and depression (94%). Persons with less incomes reported higher anxiety, which makes sense in the context of the increased costs of being away from work and home while at the hospital.[13]

Nurses can play an important role in helping family members of ICU patients be able to spend the night near the patient while ensuring that the family gets adequate sleep and rest. Frisman and colleagues suggest that nurses have health-promoting conversations with families. They emphasize the need that families have for information during the ICU stay as well as after discharge and that nurses are able to facilitate those conversations in order to help meet the family's needs.[14] Nurses can also encourage the use of diaries, which have been found by some researchers to be helpful and certainly not harmful.[15,16] Nurse-led follow-up clinics can help after discharge to continue to have those conversations about the importance of sleep and health for the caregiver/family member.[17] As previously mentioned, nurses can offer care items to families, such as ear plugs, masks, and a comfortable sleep environment that allows them to be close to the patient and yet not disturbed by routine nursing care. Nurses can emphasize a "tuck in time" where they perform sleep hygiene for the patient and encourage the family members to do the same. At this same time, nurses can assure the family member that they will be present to care for the patient and help to alleviate the family's fears that the patient may need something while they are asleep.[9]

## IMPACT ON HEALTHCARE DELIVERY/NURSING CARE

Hetland[18] describes a tridactic relationship between patient, family, and nurses. They report that the nurse, patient, family, and environment can have the potential to serve as barriers or facilitators to collaboration. This study found that nurses use their assessment skills to determine which family members are able to assist with patient care and what that care would involve. Nurses can have conversations with families and determine their desire to assist with care and be present near the bedside versus those who may prefer a more passive approach. When the nurse determines that the family member prefers to be with the patient, and may be sleeping in the ICU room, the nurse can begin the education process about the importance of sleep for both the patient and the family. Although this might add to the responsibilities of the nurse, having these crucial conversations will be best for the patient, family, and the nurses.[18]

From an ICU environment perspective, having an additional person sleeping in the room may sometimes be a barrier to providing care. Working with the family, the nurse can find a comfortable location for the family to sleep, which allows the nurse to continue to have access to all equipment and the patient.[5]

## DISCUSSION

Patients report a sense of comfort in knowing their family members are with them in the ICU.[6] Families at the bedside of an ICU patient have positive effects on both the patient and the family. There are downsides to having family at the bedside of the ICU patient, including the possible lack of sleep for the family member, increased workload for nurses, and family member physical presence in the small space of a busy ICU room.[11] Nurses can help to minimize the sleep disruptions to both the patient and the family to ensure that both experience restorative sleep. As much as possible, nurses can cluster their care and try to promote a quiet environment with less disruptions in sleep. Nurses can provide education to families about the importance of uninterrupted sleep for both the patient and family and provide both with comfort measures such as ear plugs, eye masks, and comfortable sleeping arrangements. Having the patient sleep well can improve their ability to overcome critical illness, and having the family obtain restorative sleep can help them make the important decisions that they often need to make and promote their overall comfort.[14]

Some families may find the use of an ICU diary helpful in recording what is happening on a day-to-day basis, giving them a sense of purpose and helping with feelings of anxiety.[19] If possible, family members can take turns staying overnight with the patient while others sleep at home, thus not having sleep deprivation for one person day after day. Each family will be unique in their ability to assist with patient care needs, maintain their own health while being with their loved one in the ICU, and determine if sleeping in the ICU room is the right thing to do for themselves and the patient. Nurses can assist with facilitating conversations so that the family member weighs the risks and benefits of these important decisions.[14]

## SUMMARY

Sleep is important for both the ICU patient and their family members. Patients report that having family at the bedside is important; however, there are risks to family members in terms of sleep deprivation. Nurses can help mitigate those risks by having family-centered conversations about the importance of self-care for the family member while also assisting them in being supportive and caring for the patient.

## CRITICS CARE POINTS

- ICU environments are not ideal for obtaining restorative sleep for the patient or the family members.
- Families who sleep in the ICU can be assisted with a comfortable sleep location, eye masks, and ear plugs.
- Nurses can assist with the health of the family members by educating about the importance of sleep for both the patient and the family.

## DISCLOSURE

The authors have nothing to disclose.

## REFERENCES

1. Hashemian S, Kassiri N. Sleep disorders in critical care unit. J Pulmonol Clin Res 2018;2(1):731–8.
2. Society of Critical Care Medicine. Clinical Practice Guidelines for the prevention and management of pain, agitation/sedation, delirium, immobility, and sleep disruption in adult patients in the ICU. Crit Care Med 2018;46(9):e825–73.
3. Pulak L, Jensen L. Sleep in the intensive care unit. J Intensive Care Med 2016; 31(1):14–23.
4. Ding Q, Redeker N, Pisani M, et al. Factors influencing patients' sleep in the Intensive Care Unit: Perceptions of patients and clinical staff. Am J Crit Care 2017; 26(4):278–86.
5. Netzer G. An introduction and overview into why families matter in the inetnsive care unit. In The book, Families in the intensive care unit. Springer Publishing; 2018. doi:10.1007978-3-319-94337-4.
6. Wåhlin I, Samuelsson P, Ågren S. What do patients rate as most important when cared for in the ICU and how often is this met? – an empowerment questionnaire survey. J Crit Care 2017;40:83–90.
7. McAdam J, Arai S, Puntillo K. Unrecognized contributions of families in the intensive care unit. Intensive Care Med 2008;34(6):1097–101.
8. Verceles A, Corwin D, Afshar M, et al. Half of the family members of critically ill patients experience excessive daytime sleepiness. Intensive Care Med 2014; 40(8):1124–31.
9. Meneguin S, Souza M, Ticiane D, et al. Association between comfort and needs of ICU patients' family members: a cross-sectional study. J Clin Nurs 2019; 28(3–4):538–44.
10. Owens R, Huynh TG, Netzer G. Sleep in the intensive care unit in a Model of family-centered care. AACN Adv Crit Care 2017;28(2):171–8.

11. Jaiswal S, Owens R. Sleep and sleep deprivation among families in the ICU. In: Families in the intensive care unit. Cham: Springer International Publishing; 2018. p. 61–75.
12. Choi J, Tate J, Donahoe M, et al. Sleep in family caregivers of ICU survivors for two months post-ICU discharge. Intensive Crit Care Nurs 2016;37:11–8.
13. Celic S, Genc G, Kinetli Y, et al. Sleep problems, aniety, depression and fatigue on family members of adult intensive care unit patients. Int J Nurs Pract 2016; 22(5):512–22.
14. Frisman G, Wahlin I, Orvelius L, et al. Health-promoting conversations—a novel approach to families experiencing critical illness in the ICU environment. J Clin Nurs 2018;27(3–4):631–9.
15. Garrouste-Orgeas M, Flahault C, Vinatier I, et al. Effect of an ICU diary on post-traumatic stress disorder symptoms among patients receiving mechanical ventilation: a randomized clinical trial. JAMA 2019;322(3):229–39.
16. Mickelson R, Piras S, Brown L, et al. The use and usefulness of ICU diaries to support family members of critically ill patients. J Crit Care 2021;61:168–76.
17. Jónasdóttir RJ, Klinke ME, Jónsdóttir H. Integrative review of nurse-led follow-up after discharge from the ICU. J Clin Nurs 2016;25(1–2):20–37.
18. Hetland B, McAndrew N, Perazzo J, et al. A qualitative study of factors that influence active family involvement with patient care in the ICU: survey of critical care nurses. Intensive Crit Care Nurs 2018;44:67–75.
19. Wang S, Xin H-N, Chung Lim Vico C, et al. Effect of an ICU diary on psychiatric disorders, quality of life, and sleep quality among adult cardiac surgical ICU survivors: a randomized controlled trial. Crit Care 2020;24(1):81.

Printed and bound by CPI Group (UK) Ltd, Croydon, CR0 4YY

03/10/2024

01040401-0013